# Challenges in
# Colorectal Surgery

Commissioning Editor: *Sue Hodgson*
Project Development Manager: *Rachel Robson*
Project Manager: *Matthew Oliver*
Production Controller: *Helen Sofio*
Design Direction: *Matthew Oliver*
Artwork Direction: *Mick Ruddy*

# Challenges in Colorectal Surgery

*Edited by*

**Paul B Boulos,** MS, FRCS, FRCS Ed
Professor of Surgery,
Consultant Colorectal Surgeon,
Department of Surgery,
Royal Free and University College
Medical School,
London, UK

*and*

**Steven D Wexner,** FACS, FRCS, FRCS Ed
Professor of Surgery
Ohio State University Health Sciences Center
at Cleveland Clinic Foundation;
Clinical Professor of Surgery
Department of Surgery
University of South Florida;
Chief of Staff, Cleveland Clinic Florida
Ft Lauderdale, Florida, USA

W. B. SAUNDERS

London  Edinburgh  New York  Philadelphia  St Louis  Sydney  Toronto  2000

WB SAUNDERS
An imprint of Harcourt Publishers Limited

© Harcourt Publishers Limited 2000

 is a registered trademark of Harcourt Publishers Limited

The right of Paul Boulos and Steven Wexner to be identified as authors of
this work has been asserted by them in accordance with the Copyright,
Designs and Patents Act 1988

First published 2000

ISBN 0–7020–2559–3

**British Library Cataloguing in Publication Data**
A catalogue record for this book is available from the British Library

**Library of Congress Cataloging in Publication Data**
A catalog record for this book is available from the Library of Congress

**Note**
Medical knowledge is constantly changing. As new information becomes
available, changes in treatment, procedures, equipment and the use of
drugs become necessary. The editors and the publishers have taken
care to ensure that the information given in this text is accurate and
up to date. However, readers are strongly advised to confirm that the
information, especially with regard to drug usage, complies with
the latest legislation and standards of practice.

The
Publisher's
policy is to use
**paper manufactured
from sustainable forests**

Typeset by Newgen
Printed in China

# Contents

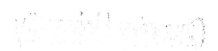

I dedicate this book to Marilyn, Mark, Sarah-Jane and Paula.

*Paul B Boulos*

I would like to dedicate my portion of the book to my children, Wesley and Trevor, and to my wife, Dr Pamela Wexner, as it was time away from them that was required to produce this work. I am indebted to them for their love, support and understanding.

*Steven D Wexner*

# Contributors

Paul B Boulos, MS, FRCS, FRCS
Professor of Surgery,
Consultant Colorectal Surgeon,
Department of Surgery,
Royal Free and University College
Medical School, London, UK

Marc I Brand, MD
Assistant Professor of Surgery,
Section of Colon and Rectal Surgery,
Department of General Surgery,
Rush Medical College,
Rush-Presbyterian-St. Luke's
Medical Center,
Chicago, Illinois, USA

James M Church FACS, FRACS, FACG
Staff Surgeon,
Department of Colorectal Surgery,
Cleveland Clinic;
Associate Professor of Surgery,
Ohio State University,
Health Sciences Center,
Cleveland Clinic;
Head of Endoscopy,
Department of Colorectal Surgery,
Director, David G Jagelman Inherited
Colorectal Cancer Registry,
Cleveland, Ohio, USA

Zane Cohen, MD, FRCS, FACS
Professor and Chairman,
Division of General Surgery,
University of Toronto;
Surgeon-in-Chief,
Mount Sinai Hospital,
Toronto, Ontario, Canada

Alice Gillams, MD
Senior Lecturer and Consultant
in Imaging and Radiology,
Department of Imaging and Radiology,
Middlesex Hospital, London, UK

Stanley M Goldberg, MD, FACS, Hon
FRACS, Hon FRCS, AFC, Hon FRCPS, Hon RSM
Clinical Professor of Surgery,
Division of Colon and Rectal Surgery,
Department of Surgery,
University of Minnesota,
Minneapolis, Minnesota, USA

Christian T Hamel, MD
Research Fellow,
Department of Colorectal Surgery,
Cleveland Clinic Florida,
Ft Lauderdale, Florida, USA

Richard E Karulf, MD, FACS, FASCRS
Associate Clinical Professor of Surgery,
Division of Colon and Rectal Surgery,
Department of Surgery,
University of Minnesota,
Minneapolis, Minnesota, USA

William R Lees, FRCR, FRACR
Professor of Imaging and Radiology
Department of Imaging and Radiology
Middlesex Hospital
London, UK

Constantinos Mavrantonis, MD
Research Fellow,
Department of Colorectal Surgery,
Cleveland Clinic Florida,
Ft Lauderdale, Florida, USA

Lars Påhlman, MD, PhD
Professor of Surgery,
Department of Sugery,
University Hospital,
Akademika Sjukhaset,
Uppsala, Sweden

Johann Pfeifer, MD
Associate Professor of Surgery,
Department of General Surgery,
Karl-Franzens University School of
Medicine,
Graz, Austria

James Pitt, MSc, FRCS
Specialist Registrar,
Bedford Hospital,
Bedford, Bedfordshire, UK

Theodore J Saclarides, MD
Professor of Surgery and Head,
Section of Colon and Rectal Surgery,
Department of General Surgery,
Rush Medical College,
Rush-Presbyterian-St. Luke's
Medical Center,
Chicago, Illinois, USA

Asha Senapati, MD, PhD, FRCS
Consultant Colorectal Surgeon,
Queen Alexandra Hospital,
Portsmouth, Hampshire, UK

Jay J Singh, MD
Staff Surgeon,
Piedmont Colorectal Associates,
Atlanta, Georgia, USA

Robert J C Steele, MD, FRCS
Professor of Surgical Oncology,
Department of Surgery,
Ninewells Hospital and
Medical Centre,
Dundee, Tayside, UK

Selman Uranüs, MD, FACS
Associate Professor of Surgery,
Department of General Surgery,
Karl-Franzens University School of
Medicine,
Graz, Austria

Steven D Wexner, MD, FACS,
FASCRS, FACG
Professor of Surgery,
Ohio State University Health Sciences
Center at Cleveland Clinic Foundation;
Clinical Professor of Surgery,
Department of Surgery,
University of South Florida;
Chief of Staff, Cleveland Clinic Florida,
Ft Lauderdale, Florida, USA

# Preface

This textbook was designed with a specific aim. We sought to address a finite number of the most controversial subjects within colorectal surgery. Rather than making this book a duplication of one of the many already available excellent comprehensive treatises on the subject, we elected to focus upon some of these controversies. The subjects were chosen to represent a variety of topics that are frequently debated both in the literature and in academic forums. In order to provide a comprehensive overview, experts were selected from the United Kingdom, continental Europe, the United States, and Canada. By doing so, this book represents the opinions of luminaries recognized for each of these specific respective topics. Authors were selected based upon their publicly acknowledged expertise within each of these subject areas as attested to by their contributions to the literature and at major meetings. One of the other advantages of focusing upon selected topics is that the book is of a very readable size. Rather than producing a voluminous tome that might become rapidly outdated, we hope to make this book the first within a series, which will cover some of the most controversial subjects within our specialty. We hope that you enjoy and learn from the labors of the contributors to this volume. We are certainly indebted to them for having taken time from their busy practices to enlighten all of us with their exchanges.

Paul B Boulos
Steven D Wexner
2000

# Acknowledgements

We wish to acknowledge the assistance and support of a number of people in the publication of this book. In particular we acknowledge our staff in our respective offices: Emma Collins, Personal Assistant to Professor Boulos at the Royal Free and University College Medical School, provided diligent help and support in the completion of the book. Elektra McDermott, Publications Manager at the Cleveland Clinic Florida, coordinated communication amongst our own offices and those of the contributors and publishers. She was also of invaluable assistance in proofreading the manuscripts and page proofs. We are also grateful to the staff at Harcourt Health Sciences, in particular Sue Hodgson and Matthew Oliver who have facilitated the processing of the book within a very tight schedule. We also acknowledge the partial support provided by a grant from the Onassis Education Foundation for the work of Constantinos Mavrantonis while at the Cleveland Clinic, and the generous support for incontinence research in the Department of Colorectal Surgery provided by the ANA Tech LLC Company.

# 1 Evidence-based surgery: pre- and postoperative care

*Jay J Singh, Christian T Hamel*
*and Steven D Wexner*

## INTRODUCTION

The irony in the pedantic search for truth is that old truths are rarely corroborated. In fact, they are typically refuted and then forsaken. The dogmatic approach to the science of medicine does have its merits, particularly in the early stages of knowledge acquisition. 'Pearls' of wisdom, many of them 'black pearls', are passed from generation to generation of physicians, with some surviving these transitions despite proof of their mendacity. It is the duty of science to scrutinize old truths, for verity is substantiated only after the appropriate questions have been asked and then answered. Dogma is that which deserves reconsideration and that which must be set in order. We, as modern scientists, then must create order by either verification or vilification. In the field of colorectal surgery, opinion rather than evidence has dominated three very important controversies that affect the general practice of this specialty. Contention continues to exist in regard to the most appropriate form of bowel preparation prior to colorectal resection, the nature and treatment of postoperative adhesions, and the necessity of postoperative nasogastric decompression and avoidance of feeding.

## BOWEL PREPARATION AND CONFINEMENT

### Mechanical bowel preparation

Since the 1950s, proper bowel cleansing has been established as a standard for elective colorectal surgery.[1,2] Furthermore, the necessity for cleansing of the bowel is obvious in diagnostic procedures such as colonoscopy, as pathology may escape detection when obscured by small particles of stool. Bowel preparation has even been encouraged in anorectal procedures, both as a means of decreasing the infectious risk inherent to colorectal surgery and of enhancing the ease and esthetics of these often complicated procedures.[3,4]

Experimental and clinical studies have shown an impact of intraluminal fecal loading on the incidence of anastomotic disruption and subsequent leakage.[5] In a randomized prospective study of 64 dogs, Ravo *et al.* studied the effect of intraluminal fecal matter at the anastomosis, both with and without peritonitis, on the healing of a colonic anastomosis. The animals were randomized into four groups: sigmoid resection with anastomosis (group I), sigmoid resection with intraluminal fecal diversion from the anastomosis (group II), induced fecal peritonitis, sigmoid resection and anastomosis (group III), and induced fecal peritonitis, sigmoid resection with intraluminal fecal diversion from the anastomosis (group IV). The results demonstrated that early anastomotic healing can occur even in the presence of peritonitis as long as the fecal matter is diverted and prevented from coming in contact with the anastomotic site.[6] In an experimental setting, O'Dwyer *et al.* studied anastomotic integrity following low anterior resection in 36 dogs randomized to either receive or forego mechanical bowel preparation. Pelvic abscess and death from peritonitis occurred in 6% of the group with bowel preparation and 29% of the unprepared group. Mechanical bowel preparation significantly enhanced anastomotic integrity and reduced complications in this model.[7]

The ideal colon evacuant should not leave fecal material or fluid behind. Several other variables have been used to compare the efficacy of bowel-cleansing regimes. These include safety, side effects, overall cost, and patients' tolerance. Furthermore, the evacuant should be easily administered in an outpatient setting.[8,9] Traditional methods for bowel cleansing have been estimated as only 70% adequate.[10,11] The emergence of polyethylene glycol (PEG) solutions essentially revolutionized mechanical bowel preparation. The process went from a tedious multiday preparation that required a hospital admission to a simple outpatient preparation that produced equivalent results. Dipalma & Marshal[12] prescribed a 4-liter PEG bowel preparation administered the day prior to operation to replace the traditional 3-day inhospital regimen. PEG solution had a satisfactory performance in both the inhospital as well as in the outpatient setting allowing most admissions to take place on the day of surgery[13,14] with considerable cost savings.[15] Surveys of practicing colorectal surgeons reveal that PEG-based solutions have become the mechanical bowel preparation of choice because of their relative ease of administration.[14] Despite the popularity achieved among surgeons, many patients find it difficult to tolerate the large volume required (4 liters), the salty taste, and the gastrointestinal side effects including abdominal distention, nausea, and cramping.[16] The incidence of these side effects approaches 100% in some series.[17–19] The overall incidence of mild gastrointestinal discomfort is 33% with a small but significant number of subjects who are unable to finish the solution. Some authors recommend the empiric, adjunctive use of metoclopramide,[20–22] while others believe its routine use is not indicated.[23]

To improve patient compliance, small volume sodium phosphate (NaP) oral solution (Fleet Phospho-Soda, CB Fleet Co.) was developed. This proved to be a superior mechanical bowel preparation to a PEG solution, as significant improvements in patient compliance and tolerance were noted.[24] In 1990, Vanner *et al.*[25] in a prospective randomized trial compared oral NaP with standard PEG-based lavage solution in the preparation of patients for colonoscopy. Endoscopists, unaware of the type of lavage solution, scored the degree of colonic cleansing significantly higher for colons prepared with NaP compared with the PEG-based lavage solution GoLYTELY. The 37 patients in this study who received oral NaP had previously received a GoLYTELY preparation for earlier procedures. All patients reported an easier consumption of the NaP solution. Also, over 90% of these patients admitted to less discomfort with the NaP preparation than they recalled with the GoLYTELY preparation. The authors concluded that NaP is a safe colonic cleansing agent that is better tolerated and, as a result, more effective than standard PEG-based lavage solution.

In 1994, Cohen *et al.*[24] studied 450 patients who underwent colonoscopy prospectively randomized to receive either a standard 4-liter PEG solution, a sulfate-free 4-liter PEG solution, or a 90-ml oral NaP preparation. Endoscopists, blinded to the preparation, scored the type of residual stool and the percentage area of bowel wall visualized for each segment of colon and for the overall examination. Based on these parameters, the NaP preparation was more effective in colon cleansing, and it was preferred by patients, who seemed to enjoy the smaller volumes and minimal side effects. The authors do mention that in patients, with impaired renal function, hyperphosphatemia may limit the use of this preparation. In order to verify the cleansing performance, patient compliance, and safety of 90 ml of NaP in comparison to 4 liters of standard PEG solution as mechanical bowel preparation for elective colorectal surgery, a prospective, randomized, surgeon-blinded trial was performed by one of the same authors;[26] 200 patients, matched for age, gender, and diagnosis, received either PEG or NaP solutions. A significant decrease in serum calcium levels after administration of both NaP and PEG could be shown. No clinical sequelae were apparent. Patient tolerance to NaP was superior to PEG, as 65% of patients who received NaP stated that they would repeat this preparation compared with only 25% for the PEG group. Ninety-five per cent of patients who received the NaP solution tolerated the entire preparation compared with only 37% of the PEG group. The quality of cleansing based on the presence of gas, fluid, particulate formed stool, or large solid stool by peroperative inspection, palpation, and proctoscopy was scored as 'excellent' or 'good' in 87% after NaP compared with 76% after PEG preparation (PNS). The rates of septic and anastomotic complications were 1% and 1% for NaP and 4% and 1% for PEG, respectively (PNS).

An unusual complication was reported by Hixson who found that NaP solution produces aphthous ulcers in the left colon, particularly in the distal sigmoid and rectum, when applied as an oral lavage solution.[27] These findings were confirmed by Zwas et al.[28] in 24% of the patients who received NaP in a randomized trial, but have been disputed by others.[24–26,29,30]

In light of superior subjective patient tolerance, comparable surgeon preference, and safety, NaP should be the standard mechanical bowel preparation for elective colorectal surgery. Other preparations may have to be considered in patients with chronic renal failure.

## Antibiotic bowel preparation

After elective colorectal surgical resection, septic complications have been reported at between 30% and 60% when antibiotic prophylaxis is not used.[31–35] This results in significant mortality and morbidity. The ongoing search for the most effective single agent or combination of antimicrobial agents to reduce these septic complications has been addressed in the literature. However the data are difficult to analyze, even in prospective randomized trials. In 1987 Evans & Pollock[36] assessed 56 papers published between 1979 and 1986 that tested regimens of antibacterial bowel preparation before elective colorectal procedures, using a numerical score. Only 13 (23%) reached a satisfactory score. The most frequent errors in design were the use of placebos in the control group (27%) and faulty methods of randomization (36%); errors in analysis included the omission of confidence limits, confusion of exclusions and withdrawals (46%), not recording the fate of withdrawals (80%), and incorrect use of statistical tests (55%). In 10 papers showing important clinical differences the results did not achieve statistical significance and only two considered type II error. Defects in presentation were less frequently encountered, the most common being inaccessibility of raw data (66%), lack of sufficient information to allow replication of methods (43%), and drawing firm conclusions from inconclusive data (50%). It was particularly disappointing that there was no evidence of improvement in the standard of these reports over the 7-year period.

Currently, the use of antibiotics in addition to mechanical cleansing is the standard of care before colonic surgery.[37–39] Support for this combined approach in North America has been shown in a survey of 352 Board Certified, active colon and rectal surgeons.[38] It is also generally agreed that the antibiotics should be active against both the aerobic and anaerobic colonic bacteria. The question whether an antibiotic has to be administered either intravenously or orally or by both routes has been and is still a topic of some debate. The importance of reducing the number of microorganisms in the colonic lumen is emphasized by the advocates of oral administration, while advocates of parenteral administration emphasize the importance of adequate tissue levels of the antibiotics. Oral nonabsorbable antibiotics serve to reduce the concentration of colonic bacteria but have little, if any, systemic effects. Systemic agents protect against the almost inevitable intraperitoneal and wound bacterial contamination that may occur at the time of surgery. It is recognized that an antibiotic, to be effective, must be at a sufficiently high tissue concentration level at the time of contamination. This concept concurs with the now accepted use of parenteral antibiotics for prophylaxis of surgical infections.[40–42] While there is almost universal agreement on the antibiotics to be employed, the route of administration has remained a topic for some debate.

### Oral antibiotics alone

The classic randomized prospective study by Clarke *et al.*[43] showed the effectiveness of oral nonabsorbable agents in decreasing the septic complications of colonic surgery using the 'Nichols–Condon' combination of erythromycin with neomycin to cover both aerobic and anaerobic bacteria. Over a decade later, Lewis *et al.*[44] compared the combination of erythromycin and neomycin with a combination of erythromycin and metronidazole. The reason behind adding metronidazole was to broaden the anaerobic cover. Fewer wound infections were noted in patients who were treated with erythromycin–metronidazole combination ($P=0.057$), and five of seven wound infections in the erythromycin–neomycin group resulted from anaerobic bacteria, while in the metronidazole group two wound infections were caused by aerobic bacteria. The study showed the true need for a broad-spectrum antianaerobic antibiotic and that neomycin was inadequate for this purpose. The timing of administration of oral agents appears to be critical,[45,46] and in this respect when surgery is delayed or is prolonged combined oral and parenteral antibiotics provide adequate tissue levels.

### Parenteral antibiotics alone

The first prospective randomized, double-blind study of parenteral antibiotic prophylaxis in elective colonic resection using intramuscular cephaloridine was published in 1969.[47] The authors reported a significant reduction of postoperative infections (30–70%) in the group of patients receiving antibiotic and mechanical preparation when compared to patients who received mechanical bowel preparation alone. By contrast, other studies using first-generation cephalosporins failed to show a benefit over placebo[48] or oral neomycin and erythromycin.[49,50] In a comparison between systemic and oral antimicrobial prophylaxis in colorectal surgery, Keighley *et al.*[51] reported a reduction in bacterial concentration in the colon with oral administration of kanamycin and metronidazole but inadequate antimicrobial tissue concentration and a significantly higher wound infection rate than when kanamycin and metronidazole were administered parenterally. A survey in 1990 revealed that parenteral antibiotics are used alone for preoperative colon preparation by fewer than 10% of actively involved colon and rectal surgeons.[38]

### Combination of oral and parenteral antibiotics

In a cooperative Veterans Administration study of the septic complication rate during large-bowel surgery, Condon *et al.*[52] studied the efficacy of oral and systemic antibiotic prophylaxis in 1128 colorectal operations. The overall septic complication rate was 7.8% in patients receiving only oral antibiotics and 5.7% in patients receiving both oral and parenteral antibiotics. This difference was not significant. The authors concluded that there was no discernible benefit from adding parenteral antibiotic prophylaxis if appropriate mechanical cleansing and oral neomycin and erythromycin therapy are employed.

Playforth *et al.*[53] conducted a randomized controlled trial in 119 consecutive patients undergoing elective colorectal operations. They compared the postoperative results in patients receiving parenteral or oral antimicrobial prophylaxis alone or a combination of oral and parenteral antibiotics. Oral bowel preparation resulted in a significantly smaller number of operative cultures of fecal gram-negative aerobes and anaerobes than did the purely parenteral regimen. The rates of infective complications were higher in the parenteral alone group than in the combined group (27.6% vs 13.9%), the difference in wound infection rates being statistically significant.

Another randomized controlled trial, from Spain,[54] compared 93 patients who received oral neomycin and erythromycin base for 24 hours before operation to a regimen of one preoperative and two postoperative parenteral doses of gentamycin and metronidazole. The total septic complication rate in the oral group was 9% compared with 35% in the parenteral group. The authors concluded that patients undergoing elective colorectal operations should receive oral as well as parenteral antimicrobial bowel preparation.

Jagelman *et al.*[55] compared oral neomycin alone to oral neomycin with additional intravenous metronidazole given perioperatively in a prospective randomized setting. The combination of oral and intravenous antibiotics showed a statistically significant decrease in septic complication rates.

In a prospective randomized study Schoetz *et al.*[56] showed that the addition of perioperative parenteral cefoxitin greatly reduced the incidence of wound infections in patients undergoing elective colorectal operations who had been prepared with mechanical bowel cleansing and oral antimicrobial agents.

Becker & Alexander[57] prospectively studied the efficacy of a short perioperative versus an extended postoperative course of intravenous antibiotics (cefoxitin) in patients undergoing colectomy with ileoanal anastomosis. Forty patients were randomized to receive extended postoperative antibiotic treatment, in addition to the preoperative oral preparation with perioperative antibiotics. No differences in overall postoperative morbidity were observed and none of the patients in either group developed intra-abdominal, pelvic, or wound infections. Going one step further to decrease the incidence of wound infection, Raahave *et al.*[58] tested the topical application of ampicillin in addition to intravenously administered cefotaxime in 193 patients undergoing elective colorectal operations. The authors found no significant differences in rates of wound dehiscence, intra-abdominal abscess, or anastomotic leakage.

In a large prospective study of 350 patients, Coppa & Eng[59] showed the association of wound infection with the length of operation and the location of colonic resection. Analysis of length of operation revealed that in operations lasting 215 minutes or more, the infection rate was 12%; in those lasting less than 215 minutes the rate was 4%. Patients with rectal resection and operative times of 215 minutes or more had a wound infection rate of 19% compared to 2% in those with shorter nonrectal operations ($P<0.05$). The authors could demonstrate a significantly lower wound infection rate with the use of a combination of oral and parenteral antibiotics.

Presently, most surgeons use both oral and parenteral antibiotic agents in addition to mechanical cleansing as preoperative preparation before elective colorectal surgery.[37,38] In 1979 a survey of more than 500 surgeons reported that systemic antibiotics were used alone by 8%, oral antibiotics alone by 37%, and a combination by 49% of the surgeons.[52] A more recent survey of over 360 colon and rectal surgeons reports that more than 88% used both oral and systemic antibiotic agents before elective colon resection. The most commonly used agents were neomycin and erythromycin and a parenterally administered second-generation cephalosporin that has both aerobic and anaerobic activity.[38]

## Bowel confinement

If decreasing the amount of stool, and hence the bacterial flora, in the colon minimizes the potential septic complications related to resection and anastomosis of bowel, it is reasonable for surgeons to assume that infectious complications could be avoided after anal reconstruction surgery using a medical colostomy, typically referred to as bowel confinement. Citing all of the implications of colostomy creation, primarily its social and economic issues, as reasons to avoid it, authors have promoted oral restriction and the use of opiates and antimotility agents to effectively direct stool from the site of recent anorectal surgery. While sound in theory, this practise was routinely applied without the evidence to support it. Earlier reports on anorectal reconstructive surgery make mere mention of this topic and focus on technical and outcome issues.[3–5]

Recently Nessim and colleagues[60] compared postoperative morbidity, cost, and tolerance in patients with and without medical bowel confinement after anorectal reconstructive procedures. Fifty-four female patients undergoing either sphincteroplasty for incontinence or transanal advancement flaps for fistulas were randomly assigned to receive either a regular diet or a bowel confinement regimen consisting of a clear liquid diet, loperamide three times daily, and codeine four times daily until the third postoperative day, at which time they were advanced to a regular diet. With regard to the overall results in these two groups, the incidence of postoperative infection was 7.4% and the functional results after a mean follow up of 13 months were identical. Unrestricted diet did not contribute to higher rates of sepsis or impaired function. Furthermore, the patients on the confinement regimen had a greater tendency to experience nausea and vomiting, a longer delay to the first bowel movement, and a higher incidence of fecal impaction. Finally, the mean cost of hospitalization in the confinement group was an average of $US2000.00 more than for the unrestricted group. Thus, the omission of bowel confinement results in quicker resumption of bowel function and overall savings without the added risk of complications.

# ADHESIONS

## Incidence and cost of adhesions

Up to 1% of all adult general surgery admissions are due to adhesions and, currently, up to 3.3% of all laparotomies are performed for adhesion-related bowel obstruction.[61] In addition, adhesions prolong and may complicate many laparotomies performed for other disease processes. After laparotomy, up to 93% of patients are reported to develop adhesions.[61,62] There are various theories on the etiopathogenesis of adhesions such as trauma, ischemia, foreign bodies, hemorrhage, or infection. Injury or inflammation in the peritoneal cavity results in a rapid deposition of fibrin, which causes adhesion of the involved surfaces to adjacent structures.[63–65] Adhesions are responsible for approximately 74% of intestinal obstructions.[66–69] After either left-sided colon or rectal surgery, adhesions have been reported in up to 25% of patients as compared to 15% after appendectomy and 9% after right colectomy. Raf[64] assessed 1477 adults with adhesions treated between 1954 and 1965. Eighty-six per cent of these individuals had undergone prior laparotomy, most commonly either appendectomy or a gynecologic procedure. In a postmortem study of 752 individuals,[65] adhesions were found in 67% of those who had undergone prior laparotomy. Ninety-one per cent of patients who had undergone colorectal surgery and 93% of patients who had undergone multiple prior operations developed intra-abdominal adhesions, compared to only 60% after exploratory laparotomy alone, and 47% after appendectomy. In the USA in 1988, costs for abdominal adhesiolysis mounted to nearly $1.2 billion.[70] Van Goor retrospectively analyzed the impact of previous laparotomies on bowel perforation at a second intervention. The risk of adhesion-related bowel perforation was 20% in this series. The number of previous laparotomies and the age of the patient were identified as independent risk factors.[71] In patients with previous surgery, on average the incision time is prolonged by 5 minutes and the division of relevant adhesions requires a mean of 19 minutes (range 0–120 minutes).[72]

The goal of adhesion prevention is to abolish or reduce the incidence, severity, and extent of adhesions while retaining normal healing and avoiding infection. Careful handling of tissue, avoiding undue dissection and overheated irrigant solutions while minimizing the trauma and ischemia produced by cautery, lasers, and retractors, are obvious initial measures for intervention.[73] Despite meticulous technique, adhesions are unavoidable. This simple fact has invoked science to seek physical and chemical methods to prevent adhesions. Although a variety of pharmacologic agents, solutions, and physical barriers have been proposed for adhesion prevention, none has been shown to be consistently effective.[74,75] Hyaluronic acid (HA) as a tissue precoating solution has been shown to protect tissue from injury and prevent adhesion development.[76] To provide an ideal mechanical barrier for reducing adhesion formation, a bioresorbable membrane of HA has been developed.

## Animal studies

In a rat cecal abrasion or sidewall injury model[77] the efficacy of HA-membrane was tested in the presence of blood and irrigation solutions, in multiple layers, and under ischemic conditions. Adhesion formation was evaluated both by the incidence and severity of adhesions. Among rats tested for adhesion formation, the treated group had a significantly larger proportion of adhesion-free animals than the untreated group. In a rabbit anastomosis model, the effect of the membrane on wound healing was tested. HA-membranes did not impair wound healing in an anastomosis and, more importantly, the substance was nontoxic, nonmutagenic, nonimmunogenic, nonpyrogenic, non-irritating, and biocompatible. The preclinical evaluation has revealed that HA-membrane is safe and effective in reducing postsurgical adhesions.

Moreira *et al.*[78] prospectively evaluated the safety of HA-membrane after bowel injury in a rabbit model. Sixty rabbits underwent laparotomy with equal distribution to one of three injury groups: creation of either three unrepaired myotomies, three repaired myotomies, or three repaired enterotomies. Thus, a total of 180 defects were created in the same anatomic positions in these 60 animals. One half of the animals in each group had the surface of the lesions covered by HA-membrane. Fourteen days after the intervention, the severity of adhesions, the presence of intra-abdominal abscesses, and the integrity of the suture lines were examined directly by an investigator blinded as to the presence of membrane and indirectly by standard radiographic isobaric contrast study to assess for leaks. The incidence of adhesions for both repaired and unrepaired myotomy sites was significantly reduced by the application of HA-membrane. The HA-membrane was not as effective in decreasing adhesions in the enterotomy group, yet it did not increase the septic mortality as shown by an equal number of leaks and abscesses in the entire group. These results confirm those of a study by Medina *et al.*, which showed that HA-membrane could be used in presence of inflammation, without impairing anastomotic integrity.[79] In this study, 64 rabbits were divided into two groups, each undergoing a complete or partial (90% anastomosis to simulate anastomotic leak) large bowel anastomosis. Half of each of the above groups were treated by wrapping HA-membrane over the anastomosis and the other half were untreated controls. These two subgroups were then further divided equally and sacrificed at either 7 or 14 days for evaluation of anastomosis integrity and strength. The average anastomotic bursting pressures did not change significantly between those groups treated with HA-membrane when compared to untreated controls at 7 or 14 days or in the complete or partial anastomosis group. Adhesion formation to the anastomosis was not impaired in either group independent of HA-membrane application.

## Human studies

In order to assess the efficacy of HA-membrane in reducing the symptoms of early postoperative bowel obstruction and safety relative to postoperative septic complication, Salum *et al.* retrospectively reviewed 100 consecutive laparotomy patients in whom HA-membrane was applied.[80] The results were compared to those of a control group consisting of a matched cohort of 100 patients who had laparotomy prior to the availability of HA-membrane. The incidence of sepsis, obstruction, or both was noted for a period of 30 days after the operation. In the HA-membrane group, five patients had early postoperative obstruction, all occurrences of which were successfully treated by nonsurgical means. In the control group, there were three bowel obstructions, two of which required surgical intervention. There were four septic complications in the HA-membrane group: two anastomotic leaks and two intra-abdominal abscesses. In the control group there were three septic sequelae (one toxic colitis, one enterocutaneous fistula, one intra-abdominal abscess, all surgically treated). Although it appears that HA-membrane failed to reduce the incidence of postoperative bowel obstruction in this study, the use of this substance may reduce the severity of adhesions and thus the frequency of early postoperative surgery for bowel obstruction.

A prospective, randomized, multicenter trial analyzing the incidence of adhesions after major abdominal operation was assessed by Becker *et al.* in 1996.[81] Total proctocolectomy and ileal pouch anal anastomosis (IPAA) with mucosectomy was performed in 183 patients with either familial adenomatous polyposis (FAP) or mucosal ulcerative colitis (MUC). At the time of ileostomy takedown, direct laparoscopy imaging of the midline assessed the grade and length of adhesions. Data were analyzed for 175 assessable patients. While only five (6%) of 90 control patients had no adhesions, 43 (51%) of 85 patients receiving HA-membrane were free of adhesions ($P < 0.001$). The mean per cent of the incision length involved was 63% in the control group, significantly greater than the 23% observed in patients who received HA-membrane ($P < 0.001$). Dense adhesions were observed in 52 (58%) of the 90 control patients, but in only 13 (15%) of the 85 receiving HA-membrane ($P < 0.0001$). Comparison of the incidence of specific adverse events between the groups did not identify a difference ($P > 0.05$). The authors were able to show that HA-membrane was able to statistically decrease the incidence, severity and number of adhesions. Thus a profound and immediately apparent reduction in adhesions may best be appreciated during reoperative surgery.

Until recently, no effective means of preventing adhesions has been available. The studies discussed support routine clinical application of HA-membranes.

## NASOGASTRIC TUBE/EARLY POSTOPERATIVE FEEDING

The dogmatic application of postoperative nasogastric tubes and the practise of keeping patients nil per os (NPO) until the adequate resumption of bowel function has caused much patient discomfort. Realizing that ileus is a mandatory component of abdominal surgery, the notion that perioral intake be avoided may make perfect teleological sense. The addition of a nasogastric tube seems equally tenable as a means of treating postoperative ileus. Other purported reasons for postoperative nasogastric suction are to avoid the distention of bowel by swallowed air in the hope of preventing nausea, vomiting and potential abdominal wound dehiscence or hernia and to decrease tension at suture lines and thus avoid anastomotic leak. Kussmaul may be credited as the first to use tube decompression in 1884 for the treatment of ileus.[82] After the development of the flexible nasogastric tube by Levin in 1921,[83] Wangensteen & Paine popularized its routine use in the 1930s.[84] Routine support of these postoperative rituals without a true scientific basis has been the rule since that time and even the American College of Surgeons has upheld the conventional employment of intestinal decompression after all gastrointestinal anastomoses.[85] In a recent survey of the members of the American Society of Colon and Rectal Surgeons, only 30% still use nasogastric tubes.[86]

Despite early retrospective reports that questioned the necessity of these traditions and the high incidence of associated complications,[87–93] routine nasogastric tube use and postoperative starvation persisted throughout the 1980s in many institutions. The first randomized trials comparing tube decompression to no tube in patients undergoing upper gastrointestinal surgeries such as cholecystectomy and vagotomy clearly proved that nasogastric decompression was unnecessary.[94–96] Similar prospective trials with colorectal resection and anastomosis soon followed and drew like conclusions.[97–100] Yet science failed to reverse or even question this dogma until external pressures forced a reappraisal of these issues. Ironically, the medical economics of the last decade and the topics of cost containment and decreasing the length of hospital stay rather than patient comfort were at the forefront of the recent re-evaluation of these deep-rooted post-operative tenets. Serendipitously, laparoscopic colorectal resection became feasible in the last decade as well. The laparoscopist's desire to prove the merits of this new technology and an actual faith in its minimal invasiveness led to the routine avoidance of nasogastric decompression as well as the early feeding of these postcolectomy patients. In a circuitous fashion, new trials were initiated in post-colectomy patients after laparotomy in order to review and, if neces-sary, revise the dogma that has persisted despite evidence of its superfluous use in the past.

This decade's measure of operative success and indicator of patient outcome is the overall length of hospital stay. In the absence of sig-nificant postoperative complications, the factors that predict the early discharge of patients are the tolerance of a solid diet and the return of bowel function as indicated by a bowel movement. Perhaps the largest prospective, randomized study looking at selective nasogastric decompression was published by Wolff and colleagues in 1989.[101] This study of 535 patients found that despite the fact that the patients without nasogastric suction experienced more nausea, vomiting, and distension, there were no significant differences in postoperative com-plications or in the length of hospital stay compared to patients with nasogastric tubes. In a 1995 follow-up study of this same patient pop-ulation, Otchy *et al.* discovered that the incidence of incisional hernia was not increased by the omission of routine decompression.[102] This further toppled the argument for the routine placement of nasogas-tric tubes. Finally, a meta-analysis of 26 trials selected by rigid inclu-sion criteria and containing 3964 patients was published by Cheatham and colleagues in 1995 to re-evaluate this issue.[103] Seventeen of these trials were randomized and prospective. The authors found significantly fewer pulmonary complications including fever, atelectasis, and pneumonia in the group of patients managed without nasogastric tubes. These and other upper and lower respira-tory complications related to nasogastric tubes have been noted by other authors.[104–106] More importantly, and despite the fact that the patients without decompression had more distension and vomiting, Cheatham[103] estimated that only one out of every 20 patients who have had some type of abdominal surgery will require a nasogastric tube. Thus, routine use of postoperative nasogastric decompression is not supported by current scientific literature.

Avoidance of early postoperative alimentation was really the precursor of the routine use of nasogastric suction. This concept has been a standard part of surgical teaching since the turn of the twentieth century.[107-109] However, advancements in the knowledge of gastrointestinal physiology has forced surgeons to reassess the rationale behind this theory. First, even the unstimulated gut produces over 6 liters/day of fluid that is handled and absorbed in the small intestine.[110] Second, neither the presence of bowel sounds nor the passage of flatus assures tolerance of oral intake; thus, their utility as a measure of feeding the postoperative gut is irrational.[111-113] Finally, early jejunostomy feeding in the traumatized patient population has proven both effective and beneficial.[114]

In a prospective, nonrandomized study carried out by Bufo *et al.*,[113] 31 of 36 patients undergoing elective colorectal resection were able to tolerate clear liquids *ad libitum* in the immediate postoperative period and were advanced to a regular diet as tolerated thereafter. As one would expect, the patients that were able to eat earlier were also discharged sooner (5.7 vs 8.0 days). Binderow *et al.* conducted a prospective randomized study on 64 consecutive patients who had had laparotomy and colon resection.[115] After laparotomy, all nasogastric tubes were removed and half of the patients (group I) were consigned to a traditional feeding regimen of a regular diet only after complete resolution of ileus as defined by movement of the bowels in the absence of nausea, vomiting, or abdominal distension. The other half of the patients (group II) started a regular diet on the first postoperative day. In both groups, the duration of postoperative ileus was nearly identical (3.6 and 3.4 days) and in the patients who avoided a nasogastric tube (26/32, 81.3%), there was a trend towards a shorter hospital stay (6.7 vs 8.0 days). In a similar study, Reissman *et al.* prospectively evaluated the safety and efficacy of early oral feeding in 80 consecutive patients who underwent elective laparotomy and bowel resection.[116] Eighty-one patients fed only after total resolution of ileus served as the control group. In the absence of bowel function there were no significant differences in the early and regular feeding groups with regard to vomiting (21% vs 14%, respectively), nasogastric tube reinsertion (11% vs 10%, respectively), length of ileus (3.8 vs 4.1 days, respectively), length of hospitalization (6.2 vs 6.8 days, respectively), or overall complications (7.5% vs 6.1%, respectively). Despite this, 79% of the patients in the early feeding group had advanced to a regular diet within 48 hours of initiating liquids. They were able to tolerate a regular diet significantly sooner than the control group (2.6 vs 5.0 days, $P < 0.0001$). Most recently, a prospective randomized trial performed by Stewart *et al.* verified the merits of early feeding.[117] Eighty per cent (32/40) of the patients in the study group tolerated advancement to a regular diet within 48 hours of their colorectal resections. This same group of patients passed flatus, had bowel movements, and was discharged significantly earlier than control patients.

In light of the evidence presented above, patients undergoing elective colorectal procedures should not routinely receive nasogastric tubes nor should postoperative alimentation be withheld while awaiting the objective return of bowel function.

## CONCLUSION

As surgeons, we would like to believe that the problems we solve and the questions we answer are done purely for the benefit of our patients. As realists, we must understand that medicine is practiced under a variety of constraints and that external forces such as governmental policy, managed care, the healthcare industry, and hospital administration combine to modify patient care. For this reason, the practice of evidence-based medicine is critical. Well-founded prospective randomized trials certainly make this a possibility, as does the implementation of standard regimens of preoperative and postoperative care. Several authors have shown that adherence to standardized clinical pathways in the perioperative care of patients undergoing major colorectal surgery can reduce the length of stay and, subsequently, the cost of hospitalization.[118–121] It is obvious that the studies discussed in this chapter prompt the surgeon to standardize the care of their patients with regard to the routine use of combined oral and intravenous antibiotics in combination with mechanical cleansing prior to colon resection. Also, evidence is continuing to mount in support of the routine application of sodium hyaluronic acid membrane for the prevention of adhesions. Finally, it is well established that the omission of nasogastric tubes with early diet advancement is safe and may lead to earlier hospital discharge. Circumspection is imperative, however, because the reflexive application of these new standards creates a new form of dogma. In an analysis of such protocols, Wexner has stated that 'although standardization is useful, it can also be counterproductive if such standardization represents the automatic gainsay of tradition rather than rising to the results of continued scientific scrutiny'.[122] It is thus the duty of every physician to re-evaluate tradition, for the true beneficiary of such resolve is the patient.

# REFERENCES

1   Ludwig KA, Condon RE. Preoperative bowel preparation. In: Cameron JL (ed) *Current Surgical Therapy,* 4th edn. Mosby-Year Book, St Louis, 1992;213–216

2   Bartlett JG, Condon RE, Gorbach SL, Clarke JS, Nichols RL, Ochi S. Veterans Administration Cooperative Study on Bowel Preparation for Elective Colorectal Operations: impact of oral antibiotic regimen on colonic flora, wound irrigation cultures and bacteriology of septic complications. *Ann Surg* 1978;**188**:249–254

3   Fielding LP, Stewart-Brown S, Blesovsky L, Kearney G. Anastomotic integrity after operations for large-bowel cancer: a multicentre study. *Br Med J* 1980; **281**(6237):411–414

4   Arnspiger RC, Helling TS. An evaluation of results of colon anastomosis in prepared and unprepared bowel. *J Clin Gastroenterol* 1988;**10**:638–641

5   Irvin TT, Goligher JC. Aetiology of disruption of intestinal anastomosis. *Br J Surg* 1973;**60**:461–464

6   Ravo B, Metwall N, Yeh J, Polansky P, Frattaroli FM. Effect of fecal loading with/without peritonitis on the healing of a colonic anastomosis: an experimental study. *Eur Surg Res* 1991;**23**:100–107

7   O'Dwyer PJ, Conway W, McDermott EW, O'Higgins SJ. Effect of mechanical bowel preparation on anastomotic integrity following low anterior resection in dogs. *Br J Surg* 1989;**76**:756–758

8   Michael KA, DiPiro JT, Bowden TA, Tedesco FJ. Whole-bowel irrigation for mechanical colon cleansing. *Clin Pharmacol* 1985;**4**:414–424

9   Dueholm S, Rubinstein E, Reipurth G. Preparation for elective colorectal surgery. A randomized, blinded comparison between oral colonic lavage and whole-gut irrigation. *Dis Colon Rectum* 1987;**30**:360–364

10  Nichols RL, Gorbach SL, Condon RE. Alteration of intestinal microflora following preoperative mechanical preparation of the colon. *Dis Colon Rectum* 1971;**14**:123–127

11  Beck DE, Fazio VW. Current preoperative bowel cleansing methods. Results of a survey. *Dis Colon Rectum* 1990;**33**:12–15

12  DiPalma JA, Marshall JB. Comparison of a new sulfate-free polyethylene glycolelectrolyte lavage solution versus a standard solution for colonoscopy cleansing. *Gastrointest Endosc* 1990;**36**:285–289

13  Beck DE, Fazio VW, Jagelman DG. Comparison of oral lavage methods for preoperative colonic cleansing. *Dis Colon Rectum* 1986;**29**:699–703

14 Beck DE, Fazio VW. Current preoperative bowel cleansing methods. Results of a survey. *Dis Colon Rectum* 1990;**33**:12–15

15 Le TH, Timmcke AE, Gathright JB Jr, Hicks TC, Opelka FG, Beck DE. Outpatient bowel preparation for elective colon resection. *South Med J* 1997;**90**:526–530

16 Mather MS, Maheshwari RK, Chadda VS *et al*. Evaluation of oral saline lavage for gastrointestinal tract radiology. *Am J Proctocol Gastroenterol* 1979;**30**:11–15

17 Chambers CE, Carter HG. Saline lavage; a rapid, safe, effective method of whole gut irrigation for bowel preparation. *South Med J* 1978;**71**:1065–1066

18 King DM, Dowes MO, Heddle RM. An alternative method of bowel preparation for barium enema. *Br J Radiol* 1979;**52**:388–389

19 Glass RL, Winship DH, Rogers WA. Comparison of intragastric infusion with conventional mechanical bowel preparation. *Dis Colon Rectum* 1981; **24**:589–591

20 Minervini S, Alexander-Willians J, Donavan IA *et al*. Comparison of three methods of whole bowel irrigation. *Am J Surg* 1980;**140**:400–402

21 Goldman J, Reichlderfer M. Evaluation of rapid colonoscopy preparation using a new gut lavage solution. *Gastrointest Endosc* 1982;**28**:9–11

22 Rhodes JB, Engstrom J, Stone KF. Metaclopramide reduces the distress associated with colon cleaning by an oral electrolyte overload. *Gastrointest Endosc* 1978;**24**:162–163

23 Ernstoff JJ, Howard DA, Marshall JB *et al*. A randomized blinded clinical trial of a rapid colonic lavage solution (Golytely) compared with the standard preparation for colonoscopy and barium enema. *Gastroenterology* 1983;**84**:1512–1516

24 Cohen SM, Wexner SD, Binderow SR *et al*. Prospective, randomized, endoscopic-blinded trial comparing precolonoscopy bowel cleansing methods. *Dis Colon Rectum* 1994;**37**:689–696

25 Vanner SJ, MacDonald PH, Paterson WG, Prentice RS, Da Costa LR, Beck IT. A randomized prospective trial comparing oral sodium phosphate with standard polyethylene glycol-based lavage solution (Golytely) in the preparation of patients for colonoscopy. *Am J Gastroenterol* 1990;**85**:422–427

26 Oliveira L, Wexner SD, Daniel N *et al*. Mechanical bowel preparation for elective colorectal surgery. A prospective, randomized, surgeon-blinded trial comparing sodium phosphate and polyethylene glycol-based oral lavage solutions. *Dis Colon Rectum* 1997;**40**:585–591

27 Hixson LJ. Colorectal ulcers associated with sodium phosphate catharsis. *Gastrointest Endosc* 1995;**42**:101–102

28 Zwas FR, Cirillo NW, el-Serag HB, Eisen RN. Colonic mucosal abnormalities associated with oral sodium phosphate solution. *Gastrointest Endosc* 1996;**43**:463–466

29 Kolts BE, Lyles WE, Achem SR, Burton L, Geller AJ, MacMath T. A comparison of the effectiveness and patient tolerance of oral sodium phosphate, castor oil, and standard electrolyte lavage for colonoscopy or sigmoidoscopy preparation. *Am J Gastroenterol* 1993;**88**:1218–1223

30 Marshall JB, Pineda JJ, Barthel JS, King PD. Prospective, randomized trial comparing sodium phosphate solution with polyethylene glycol-electrolyte lavage for colonoscopy preparation. *Gastrointest Endosc* 1993;**39**:631–634

31 Everett NT, Brogan TD, Nettleton J. The place of antibiotics in colonic surgery: a clinical study. *Br J Surg* 1969;**56**:679

32   Gordan HE, Gayloard W, Richmond DM *et al*. Operations on the colon. The role of antibiotics in preoperative preparation. *Calif Med* 1965;**103**:243

33   Leight DA. Clinical importance of infections due to *Bacteroides fragilis* and role of antibiotic therapy. *Br Med J* 1974;**3**(925):225–228

34   Vallance S, Jones B, Arabi Y, Keighley MRB. Importance of adding neomycin to metronidazole for bowel preparation. *J R Soc Med* 1983;**73**:238–240

35   Willis AT, Ferguson IR, Jones PH *et al*. Metronidazole in prevention and treatment of bacteroides infections in elective colonic surgery. *Br Med J* 1977;**1**(6061):607–610

36   Evans M, Pollock AV. The inadequacy of published random control trials of antibacterial prophylaxis in colorectal surgery. *Dis Colon Rectum* 1987;**30**:743–746

37   Nichols RL. Bowel preparation. In: Meakins JL (ed) *Surgical Infections. Diagnosis and treatment. III Prevention of infections*. Scientific American Medicine, New York, 1994;151–159

38   Solla JA, Rothenberger DA. Preoperative bowel preparation. A survey of colon and rectal surgeons. *Dis Colon Rectum* 1990;**33**:154–159

39   Gorbach SL, Condon RE, Conte Jr JE *et al*. General guidelines for the evaluations of new antiinfective drugs for prophylaxis of surgical infections – evaluations of new anti-infective drugs for surgical prophylaxis. *Clin Infect Dis* 1992;**15** (suppl 1):S313–S338

40   Miles AA, Miles EM, Burke J. The value and duration of defense reactions of the skin to the primary lodgment of bacteria. *Br J Exp Pathol* 1957;**38**:79–96

41   Burke JF. The effective period of preventive antibiotic action in experimental incisions and dermal lesions. *Surgery* 1961;**50**:161–168

42   Polk HC, Miles AA. The decisive period in the primary infection of muscle by *Escherichia coli*. *Br J Exp Pathol* 1973;**54**:99–109

43   Clarke JS, Condon RE, Bartlett JG *et al*. Preoperative oral antibiotics reduce septic complications of colon operations: results of prospective, randomized double blind clinical study. *Ann Surg* 1977;**186**:251

44   Lewis RT, Goodall RG, Marien B, Lloyd-Smith W, Park M, Wiegand FM. Is neomycin necessary for bowel preparation in surgery of the colon? Oral neomycin plus erythromycin versus erythromycin-metronidazole. *Can J Surg* 1989;**32**:265–270

45   Nicols RL, Condon RE, DiSanto AR. Preoperative bowel preparation. Erythromycin base serum and fecal levels following oral administration. *Arch Surg* 1977;**112**:1493–1496

46   DiPiro JT, Patrias JM, Townsend RJ *et al*. Oral neomycin sulfate and erythromycin base before colon surgery: a comparison of serum and tissue concentrations. *Pharmacotherapy* 1985;**5**:91–94

47   Polk HC Jr, Lopez-Mayor JF. Postoperative wound infection: a prospective study of determinant factors and prevention. *Surgery* 1969;**66**:97–103

48   Evans C, Pollock AV. The reduction of surgical wound infections by prophylactic parenteral cephaloridine. A controlled clinical trial. *Br J Surg* 1973;**60**:434–437

49   Condon RE, Bartlett JG, Nichols RL, Schulte WJ, Gorbach SL, Ochi S. Preoperative prophylactic cephalothin fails to control septic complications of colorectal operations: results of controlled clinical trial. A Veterans Administration cooperative study. *Am J Surg* 1979;**137**:68–74

50  Edmondson HT, Rissing JP. Prophylactic antibiotics in colon surgery. *Arch Surg* 1983;**118**:227–231

51  Keighley MR, Arabi Y, Alexander-Williams J, Youngs D, Burdon DW. Comparison between systemic and oral antimicrobial prophylaxis in colorectal surgery. *Lancet* 1979;**i**:894–897

52  Condon RE, Bartlett JG, Greenlee H *et al*. Efficacy of oral and systemic antibiotic prophylaxis in colorectal operations. *Arch Surg* 1983;**118**:496–502

53  Playforth MJ, Smith GM, Evans M, Pollock AV. Antimicrobial bowel preparation. Oral, parenteral, or both? *Dis Colon Rectum* 1988;**31**:90–93

54  Figueras-Filip J, Basilio-Bonet E, Lara-Eisman F *et al*. Oral is superior to systemic antibiotic prophylaxis in operations upon the colon and rectum. *Surg Gynecol Obstet* 1984;**158**:359–362

55  Jagelman DG, Fazio VW, Lavery IC, Weakley FL. A prospective, randomized, double-blind study of 10% mannitol mechanical bowel preparation combined with oral neomycin and short-term, perioperative, intravenous Flagyl as prophylaxis in elective colorectal resections. *Surgery* 1985;**98**:861–865

56  Schoetz DJ Jr, Roberts PL, Murray JJ, Coller JA, Veidenheimer MC. Addition of parenteral cefoxitin to regimen of oral antibiotics for elective colorectal operations. A randomized prospective study. *Ann Surg* 1990;**212**:209–212

57  Becker JM, Alexander DP. Colectomy, mucosal proctectomy, and ileal pouch–anal anastomosis. A prospective trial of optimal antibiotic management. *Ann Surg* 1991;**213**:242–247

58  Raahave D, Hesselfeldt P, Pedersen T, Zachariassen A, Kann D, Hansen OH. No effect of topical ampicillin prophylaxis in elective operations of the colon or rectum. *Surg Gynecol Obstet* 1989;**168**:112–114

59  Coppa GF, Eng K. Factors involved in antibiotic selection in elective colon and rectal surgery. *Surgery* 1988;**104**:853–858

60  Nessim A, Wexner SD, Agachan F *et al*. Is bowel confinement necessary after anorectal reconstructive surgery? A prospective randomized surgeon blinded trial. *Dis Colon Rectum* 1999;**42**:16–23

61  Menzies D, Ellis H. Intestinal obstruction from adhesions – how big is the problem? *Ann R Coll Surg Engl* 1990;**72**:60–63

62  Menzies D. Peritoneal adhesions. Incidence, cause, and prevention. *Surg Annu* 1992;**24**(Pt 1):27–45

63  Scott-Coombes C, Thompson JN, Vipond MN. General surgeon's attitudes to the treatment and prevention of abdominal surgery. *Am J Surg* 1973;**126**:345–353

64  Raf LE. Causes of abdominal adhesions in cases of intestinal obstruction. *Acta Chir Scand* 1969;**35**:73–76

65  Weibel MA, Majno G. Peritoneal adhesions and their relation to abdominal surgery. A postmortem study. *Am J Surg* 1973;**126**:345–353

66  Playforth RH, Holloway JB, Griffen WO Jr. Mechanical small bowel obstruction: a plea for earlier surgical intervention. *Ann Surg* 1970;**171**:783–788

67  Laws HL. Management of small bowel obstruction. *Am Surg* 1978;**44**:313–317

68  Stewardson RH, Bombeck CT, Nyhus LM. Critical operative management of small bowel obstruction. *Ann Surg* 1978;**187**:189–193

69  Bizer LS, Liebling RW, Delany HM, Gliedman ML. Small bowel obstruction: the role of nonoperative treatment in simple intestinal obstruction and predictive criteria for strangulation obstruction. *Surgery* 1981;**89**:407–413

70  Ray NF, Larsen JW Jr, Stillman RJ, Jacobs RJ. Economic impact of hospitalizations for lower abdominal adhesiolysis in the United States in 1988. *Surg Gynecol Obstet* 1993;**176**:271–276

71  Van Goor H. *International Society of University Colon and Rectal Surgeons, XVIIth Biennial Congress, June 7–11; Malmö, Sweden*

72  Moran BJ. *International Society of University Colon and Rectal Surgeons, XVIIth Biennial Congress, June 7–11; Malmö, Sweden*

73  Holmdahl L, Risberg B. Adhesions: prevention and complications in general surgery. *Eur J Surg* 1997;**163**:169–174

74  diZerega GS. Contemporary adhesion prevention. *Fertil Steril* 1994; **61**:219–235

75  The Surgical Membrane Study Group. Prophylaxis of pelvic sidewall adhesions with Gore-Tex surgical membrane: a multicenter clinical investigation. *Fertil Steril* 1992;**57**:921–923

76  Burns JW, Skinner K, Colt J *et al*. Prevention of tissue injury and postsurgical adhesions by precoating tissues with hyaluronic acid solutions. *J Surg Res* 1995;**59**:644–652

77  Burns JW, Colt MJ, Burgees LS, Skinner KC. Preclinical evaluation of Seprafilm bioresorbable membrane. *Eur J Surg* 1997;**577**(suppl):40–48

78  Moreira H Jr, Wexner SD, Yamaguchi T, *et al*. Use of bioresorbable membrane (sodium hyaluronate + carboxymethylcellulose) after controlled bowel injuries in a rabbit model. *Dis Colon Rectum* 2000;**43**:182–7

79  Medina M, Paddock HN, Connolly RJ, Schwaitzberg SD. Novel antiadhesion barrier does not prevent anastomotic healing in a rabbit model. *J Invest Surg* 1995;**8**:179–186

80  Salum M, Lam D, Wexner SD, *et al*. Does bioresorbable membrane of modified sodium hyaluronate and carboxymethylcellulose (Seprafilm®) have possible short term beneficial impact? *Dis Colon Rectum* (in press)

81  Becker JM, Dayton MT, Fazio VW *et al*. Prevention of postoperative abdominal adhesions by a sodium hyaluronate-based bioresorbable membrane: a prospective, randomized, double-blind multicenter study. *J Am Coll Surg* 1996;**183**:297–306

82  Kussmaul CA. Heilung von ileus durch magenausspulung. *Berl Klin Wochenschr* 1884;**21**:669–685

83  Levin AL. A new gastroduodenal catheter. *JAMA* 1921;**76**:1007–1008

84  Wangesteen OH, Paine JR. Treatment of acute intestinal obstruction by suction with the duodenal tube. *JAMA* 1993;**101**:1532–1539

85  Welch CE. In: Whinney JM (ed) *American College of Surgeons Manual of Preoperative and Postoperative Care.* WB Saunders, Philadelphia, 1971;414–424

86  Golub RW, Cirocco WC, Golub R. Current trends in gastric decompression: a survey of the American Society of Colon and Rectal Surgeons. *Dis Colon Rectum* 1994;**37**:48

87  Eade GG, Methany D, Lundmark VO. An evaluation of the practice of routine postoperative nasogastric suction. *Surg Gynecol Obstet* 1955;**101**:275–279

88  Sprong DH, Pollock WF. A reappraisal of the routine use of nasogastric suction. *Am J Surg* 1957;**94**:257–261

89  Gerber A, Rogers FA, Smith LL. The treatment of paralytic ileus without the use of gastrointestinal suction. *Surg Gynecol Obstet* 1958;**107**:247–250

90  Thomas GI, Metheny D, Lundmark VO. Vagotomy without postoperative nasogastric suction. *Northwest Med* 1961;**60**:387–391

91  Hendry WG. Tubeless gastric surgery. *Br Med J* 1962;**1**:1736–1737

92  Herrington JL, Edwards WH, Sawyers JL. Elimination of routine use of gastric decompression following operation for gastroduodenal ulcer. *Ann Surg* 1964;**159**:808–818

93  Herrington JL. Methods of postoperative decompression including an experience with the omission of its routine use. *Am J Surg* 1995;**110**:423–429

94  Miller DF, Mason JR, McArthur J, Gordon I. A randomized prospective trial comparing three established methods of gastric decompression after vagotomy. *Br J Surg* 1972;**59**:605–608

95  Edlund G, Gedda S, Van der Linden W. Intraperitoneal drains and nasogastric tubes in elective cholecystectomy: a controlled clinical trial. *Am J Surg* 1979;**137**:775–779

96  Adekunle DO, Solanke TF, Itayemi SO, Banigo OG. Tubeless postoperative care of elective cases of duodenal ulcer: A controlled study of 170 cases. *Afr J Med Sci* 1979;**8**:85–88

97  Olesan KL, Birch M, Bardram L, Burcharth F. Value of nasogastric tube after colorectal surgery. *Acta Chir Scand* 1984;**150**:251–253

98  Reasbeck PG, Rice ML, Herbison GP. Nasogastric intubation after intestinal resection. *Surg Gynecol Obstet* 1984;**158**:557–560

99  Colvin DB, Lee W, Eisenstadt TE *et al*. The role of naso-intestinal intubation in elective colonic surgery. *Dis Colon Rectum* 1986;**29**:295–299

100  Racette DL, Chang FC, Trekell ME, Farha CJ. Is nasogastric intubation necessary in colon operations? *Am J Surg* 1987;**154**:640–642

101  Wolff BG, Pemberton JH, van Heerden JA *et al*. Elective colon and rectal surgery without nasogastric decompression. A prospective, randomized trial. *Ann Surg* 1989;**209**:670–673

102  Otchy DP, Wolff BG, Van Heerden JA *et al*. Does the avoidance of nasogastric decompression following elective abdominal colorectal surgery affect the incidence of incisional hernia? *Dis Colon Rectum* 1995;**38**:604–608

103  Cheatham ML, Chapman WC, Key SP, Sawyers JL. A meta-analysis of selective versus routine nasogastric decompression after elective laparotomy. *Ann Surg* 1995;**221**:469–478

104  Schlenker JD, Hubay CA. The pathogenesis of postoperative atelectasis: a clinical study. *Arch Surg* 1973;**107**:846–850

105  Desmond P, Raman R, Idikula J. Effect of nasogastric tubes on the nose and maxillary sinus. *Crit Care Med* 1991;**19**:509–511

106  Sofferman RA, Haisch CE, Kirchner JA, Hardin NJ. The nasogastric tube syndrome. *Laryngoscope* 1990;**100**:962–968

107  Van Bergmann E, Von Bruns P, Von Mikulicz J. *System of Practical Surgery of the Alimentary Tract*. Lea Bros and Co, New York, 1904

108 Christopher F. *Textbook of Surgery*. WB Saunders, Philadelphia, 1936

109 Dacosts JC. *Modern Surgery*, 10th edn. WB Saunders, Philadelphia, 1931

110 Hessou O, Larsen RK, Sondergaard K. Improved early alimentation after radical hysterectomies without the traditional use of stomach tube. *Acta Obstet Gynecol Scand* 1988;**67**:225–228

111 Clevers GJ, Smout JP. The natural course postoperative ileus following abdominal surgery. *Neth J Surg* 1989;**41**:97–99

112 Moss G. Postoperative ileus in an avoidable complication. *Surg Gynecol Obstet* 1989;**148**:81–82

113 Bufo AJ, Feldman S, Daniels GA, Lieberman RC. Early postoperative feeding. *Dis Colon Rectum* 1994;**37**:1260–1265

114 Moore EE, Moore FA. Immediate enteral nutrition following multi-system trauma: a decade perspective. *J Am Coll Nutr* 1991;**10**:633–648

115 Binderow SR, Cohen SM, Wexner SD, Nogueras JJ. Must early postoperative oral intake be limited to laparoscopy? *Dis Colon Rectum* 1994;**37**:584–589

116 Reissman P, Teoh TA, Cohen SM, Weiss EG, Nogueras JJ, Wexner SD. Is early oral feeding safe after elective colorctal surgery? A prospective randomized trial. *Ann Surg* 1995;**222**:73–77

117 Stewart BT, Woods RJ, Collopy BT *et al*. Early feeding after elective open colorectal resections: a prospective randomized trial. *Aust NZ J Surg* 1998;**68**:125–128

118 Bradshaw BG, Liu SS, Thirlby RC. Standardized perioperative care protocols and reduced length of stay after colon surgery. *J Am Coll Surg* 1998;**186**:501–506

119 Moinische S, Bulow S, Hesselfeldt P *et al*. Convalescence and hospital stay after colonic surgery with balanced analgesia, early oral feeding, and enforced mobilisation. *Eur J Surg* 1995;**161**:283–288

120 Archer SB, Burnett RJ, Flesch LV *et al*. Implementation of a clinical pathway decreases length of stay and hospital charges for patients undergoing total colectomy in ileal pouch/anal anastomosis. *Surgery* 1997;**122**:699–705

121 Choi J, O'Connell TX. Safe and effective early postoperative feeding and hospital discharge after open colon resection. *Am Surg* 1996;**62**:853–856

122 Wexner SD. Standardized perioperative care protocols in reduced lengths of stay after colon surgery. *J Am Coll Surg* 1998;**186**:589–593(editorial)

# 2 Why is the loop ileostomy superior to the loop colostomy?

*Richard E Karulf and Stanley M Goldberg*

## INTRODUCTION

The question of when and how to divert the fecal stream is one of the most important decisions in colon and rectal surgery. The aim of temporary fecal diversion is to protect a vulnerable anastamosis or segment of bowel with an ostomy that is both easy to manage and reverse. Opinions on the best course to achieve this aim differ widely among respected authors. However, the view that a loop ileostomy is superior to transverse loop colostomy for fecal diversion is one that is easily defended.

## OSTOMY FORMATION

### Indications

Diverting intestinal stomas are created by a wide range of specialists for a large number of different procedures. The initial indication for diverting ileostomy was as a permanent end stoma as the sole procedure for acute ulcerative colitis.[1] However, early use of diverting ileostomy produced unsatisfied patients as a result of leakage from around the stoma appliance. The dissatisfaction with ileostomy extended to its application for fecal diversion, initally making the loop colostomy the ostomy of choice. In fact, only 30 years ago, 74% of ileostomates had skin problems compared with only 47% of colostomates.[2] Since that time, innovations in ostomy appliances and the availability of enterostomal therapy nurses have greatly improved patient satisfaction with all types of ostomies.[3]

Current indications for diverting stomas include protection of low colonic anastamosis, colonic or ileal pouch–anal anastamosis, and sphincter reconstruction as an alternative to resection in certain select cases of colonic perforation due to trauma, iatrogenic injury, or diverticular disease.

Ileostomy alone is not indicated for patients with distal colonic obstruction, because a competent ileocecal valve would prevent decompression of the colon and increase the possibility of a closed loop obstruction. Similarly, when diversion is required because of distal colonic or rectal perforation in patients with unprepared bowel, colostomy may be preferred to theoretically reduce the amount of stool remaining in the bowel proximal to the perforation. In these situations, it may be desirable to either intraoperatively irrigate any remaining stool in the distal limb and/or to create an ileostomy to limit subsequent contamination.

## Morbidity and mortality

Evaluating or contrasting the outcome of two similar procedures appears to be an easy task. However, the number of subtle factors that are involved in selecting the type of diverting ostomy makes comparison of retrospective series meaningless. An abbreviated list of factors to consider includes the timing of surgery (elective or emergent), any associated comorbidity, body habitus and primary preoperative diagnosis, operative findings and procedure performed, and the expertise of the surgeon creating the stoma. For example, in a retrospective study at Cook County Hospital ostomies created during elective procedures by colon and rectal surgeons were associated with a much lower complication rate than were those created by general surgeons during emergency procedures (Table 2.1).[4]

**Table 2.1** Morbidity per number of total cases based on type of procedure and specialty of surgeon (Pearl *et al.*[4])

|  | Created by colon and rectal surgeons | | Created by general surgeons | |
| --- | --- | --- | --- | --- |
|  | No. | % | No. | % |
| Transverse loop colostomy | 1/22 | (4.5) | 32/155 | (20.6) |
| Ileostomy with mucous fistula | 1/6 | (16.6) | 32/71 | (45) |
| Loop ileostomy | 0/1 | (0) | 1/5 | (20) |
| Colostomy with mucous fistula | 1/12 | (8.3) | 12/25 | (48) |

The few prospective randomized studies that have been performed reveal remarkably similar morbidity and mortality rates for loop ileostomies and loop colostomies (Table 2.2).[5–9] While outcome measurements were similar for the two types of ostomy in each study, they were different for the same type of ostomy between studies. These differences can be attributed to the unique patient populations and entry requirements in each study.

## SATISFACTION WITH OSTOMY

Patients and surgeons consider different factors when describing satisfaction with ostomies. Surgeons value safety and effectiveness, while patients are more concerned with function and convenience. The decision regarding the type of ostomy must result from balancing these and other factors for the individual patient.

### Diversion

One of the most important factors in creating fecal diversion is the efficiency in preventing the passage of stool distal to the ostomy; success of diversion of a nonretracted loop ileostomy is almost certain. In a review of 34 patients with loop ileostomy after ileal pouch–anal anastomosis, all 10 patients with stoma retraction had spillover into the distal limb while the remaining 24 patients without retraction had none.[10]

Direct comparison of the efficiency of diversion between the two types of stoma is difficult and is based largely upon subjective opinions. One study attempted to provide objective data to answer this debate by comparing five ileostomy and five colostomy patients after ingestion of a capsule containing $1 \mu Ci$ [$^{51}Cr$]sodium chromate and $500 mg$ of carmine dye.[5] The effluent from the stoma and urine were collected continuously until 24 hours had passed since all traces of the dye had disappeared from the feces. The distal colon was washed with saline and the effluent was collected from the rectum. The radioactivity of the stoma effluent, urine and distal colon washings was measured. In order to determine if there was any $^{51}Cr$ remaining in the body, whole-body counts were performed before and after ingestion of the isotope and again after the distal washings. There was minimal $^{51}Cr$ in the urine in both groups, indicating negligible absorption. There was also minimal $^{51}Cr$

**Table 2.2** Summary of stoma creation and closure morbidity

| | Study | | | | |
|---|---|---|---|---|---|
| | Gooszen et al.[6] | Khoury et al.[7] | Chen & Stuart[8] | Rutegard & Dahlgren[9] | Williams et al.[5] |
| Colostomy creation morbidity | | | | | |
| No. | 1/39 | 18/29 | — | — | 12/23 |
| % | 2.5 | 62 | — | — | 52.1 |
| Colostomy creation mortality | | | | | |
| No. | 1/39 | — | — | — | 4/24 |
| % | 2.5 | — | — | — | 16.6 |
| Ileostomy creation morbidity | | | | | |
| No. | 9/37 | 11/32 | — | — | 7/23 |
| % | 24.3 | 34.3 | — | — | 30.4 |
| Ileostomy creation mortality | | | | | |
| No. | 5/37 | — | — | — | 3/23 |
| % | 13.5 | — | — | — | 13.0 |
| Colostomy closure morbidity | | | | | |
| No. | 3/32 | — | 12/38 | — | 6/20 |
| % | 9.3 | — | 31.5 | — | 30 |
| Colostomy closure mortality | | | | | |
| No. | 0/32 | — | — | — | 0/20 |
| % | 0 | — | — | — | 0 |
| Ileostomy closure morbidity | | | | | |
| No. | 8/29 | — | 22/72 | — | 1/20 |
| % | 27.5 | — | 30.5 | — | 5 |
| Ileostomy closure mortality | | | | | |
| No. | 2/29 | — | — | — | 0/20 |
| % | 6.8 | — | — | — | 0 |
| Colostomy stoma related complications | | | | | |
| No. | 40/38 | — | 10/38 | 5/17 | 11/19 |
| % | 105 | — | 26.3 | 29.4 | 57.8 |
| Ileostomy stoma related complications | | | | | |
| No. | 30/32 | — | 13/72 | 8/32 | 3/17 |
| % | 93.7 | — | 18 | 25 | 17.6 |

recovered in distal washings from either ostomy group. However, two of the five patients in the colostomy group but none in the ileostomy group had 8 and 14%, respectively, of the isotope measured by whole-body counting after the washing had been completed. It was calculated that as there was no isotope measured in the washings, $^{51}$Cr was retained in the proximal colon from spillover. This study provides evidence of the effectiveness of the loop ileostomy in fecal diversion and therefore should influence surgeons' preference.

## Leakage

While success of fecal diversion is crucial to surgeons, a low incidence of leakage from around the ostomy is essential for patient satisfaction. Historically, patients with a transverse loop colostomy had a lower leak rate due to the thicker consistency of the stool. With improvements in ostomy creation and stoma therapy, leakage from around the appliance is now a much less frequent occurrence with a loop ileostomy than with a transverse loop colostomy. Chen & Stuart noted that 58% of patients with transverse loop colostomy complained of several problems including bleeding, prolapse, skin excoriation and leakage with the management of their ostomy compared with 18% of patients with loop ileostomy.[8] The majority of the reports for individual complications show a trend that favors loop ileostomy but the differences were not statistically significant. One report noted statistically fewer stoma appliance changes by patients with loop ileostomy compared to those individuals with loop colostomy.[5]

## Odor

Patient embarrassment about an ostomy is related as much to the odor of the stool as it is to the fear of leakage. The difference in odor between the two types of diverting ostomies is related to the amount and type of bacteria in the stool. Comparison of normal flora of ileostomy and transverse colon effluents shows a distribution of aerobic bacteria similar to that in feces. However, the ratio of anaerobes to aerobes for feces is 1000 : 1, 10 : 1 for transverse colostomy effluent, and 1 : 1000 for ileostomy effluent.[11] Just as there is an increase in the ratio of anaerobes in the colon compared to the terminal ileum, there is an increase in the total number of bacteria. The number of colony-forming units per milliliter of bacteria increases sharply from $10^7$ to $10^9$ in the terminal ileum to $10^{11}$ to $10^{12}$ just across the ileocecal valve in the cecum.

The fact that transverse colostomy effluent is more similar to feces than ileostomy effluent may in part explain why less odor is reported in patients with an ileostomy ($P < 0.01$).[5] In the series by Williams *et al.*, 13 of 20 patients with colostomy complained of odor 3 weeks after surgery but no patients with ileostomy ($n = 19$) complained during follow up. Again, this benefit can be well appreciated by patients and should be considered in the decision-making process.

## Prolapse

Prolapse of the ostomy, although less common than leakage from around the stoma appliance, is another complication that interferes with patients' satisfaction. However, the true incidence is unknown because data regarding the incidence of prolapse are rarely reported for temporary ostomies. Nonetheless, at least subjectively, many authors feel that a loop ileostomy is less prone to prolapse than is a transverse loop colostomy.[12] In one report, 76 patients were randomized into one of two groups: 37 loop ileostomies and 39 transverse loop colostomies.[6] Only one of the 32 patients (3.1%) with a loop ileostomy had prolapse during follow up compared with 16 of 38 patients (42%) with transverse loop colostomy ($P < 0.01$). The prolapse was significant enough to require modification or adaptation of the clothing of all the 16 colostomy patients. The increased incidence of prolapse after loop colostomy mitigates against creating this type of stoma.

## Fluid and electrolyte disturbance

The normally functioning ileostomy produces between 500 and 800 ml of effluent per day. Although more than 90% of the effluent is water, the average patient losses are 55 mEq (mmol) of sodium, 20 mEq (mmol) of potassium, 8 mEq (mmol) of magnesium, and 150 mg of phosphorus.[13] Almost all ileostomy patients show some signs of salt and water depletion. There is some adaptation of the ileum with time, as attested to by progressively decreased ostomy output. However, nearly all patients with an ileostomy are found to have low urinary sodium excretion and elevated blood levels of renin and aldosterone.[14] A consequence of the chronic mild dehydration is an increase in the rate of nephrolithiasis, from 3.8% in the general population to 7–18% for ileostomy patients.

When ileostomy output exceeds 1 liter per day, rapid dehydration and severe hyponatremia can occur. Common causes for ileostomy diarrhea include partial intestinal obstruction, inflammatory bowel disease, intra-abdominal infection, previous resection of small bowel, and proximal location of an ileostomy. The metabolic consequences of prolonged ileostomy diarrhea include hypokalemia and hypo-magnesemia, both of which can result in fatal arrhythmia. In spite of this theoretical problem, few reports suggest that fluid and electrolyte considerations should preclude the use of ileostomy for temporary or permanent fecal diversion.

## Obstruction

Bowel obstruction is a common complication in both forms of fecal diversion but appears to be more common with loop ileostomy. In one series of 203 consecutive loop ileostomies, bowel obstruction requiring surgery was reported in 12 of 203 patients (6%).[12] This result is similar to another large series of 117 patients with loop ileostomy in which there was a 5% obstruction rate.[15] By contrast, bowel obstruction associated with diverting loop colostomy appears to occur in only about 1% of patients.[7] However, one must be cognizant that the reason for the possible difference may be related to the different indications for their creation. A loop ileostomy is most frequently performed as an adjunct to either a total abdominal colectomy or a restorative proctocolectomy. These procedures have the highest incidence of small bowel obstruction of any intra-abdominal procedures.[16] Moreover, the theoretical tethering among the duodenojejunal flexure, the stoma and the pouch may encourage such blockage. Therefore, it may be the surgical procedure performed rather than the type of diversion selected which correlates with rates of bowel obstruction.

## Return of bowel function

Because length of stay (and therefore hospital cost) is related to the return of bowel function, it is an important factor to take into account. In a prospective randomized study of 61 patients (32 loop ileostomy and 29 transverse loop colostomy), the median number of days until first stoma action for the ileostomy group was 2.0 days (range of 1–7), while the median for the colostomy group was 4.5 days ($P < 0.001$).[7] This factor is clearly in favor of the loop ileostomy.

## CLOSURE OF OSTOMY

### Morbidity and mortality

Loop ileostomies and colostomies have been closed without a laparotomy with a low complication rate in several reports.[12,17] In these series, the 2% complication rate for ileostomy closure (anastomotic leak, mechanical obstruction, wound infection) was similar to the 5% complication rate for loop colostomy closure (extramural hematoma, pneumonia, incisional hernia). Colostomy closure has been associated with a high complication rate (23.9% overall) when all forms of colostomy are considered.[18] This is partly due to the inclusion of late complications (midline hernias and death due to metastatic colon cancer), which were not considered in other series. The early complication rate (15.2%) similar to other reports included cerebrovascular accident, pneumonia, prolonged ileus, anastamotic leak, and pulmonary embolus. In several series, when only transverse loop colostomy was compared with loop ileostomy, there were no differences in stoma-related complications or closure rates between the two groups,[7–9] except for the infection rate which after ileostomy closure (0%) is significantly less ($P < 0.05$) than after colostomy closure (30%).[5] This is an advantage in favor of loop ileostomy.

### 'Temporary' versus permanent ostomy

Although designed as a temporary diversion for the fecal stream, not all patients elect to or can have their ostomies closed. The wide range in closure rates seems to indicate that both patient factors and the indications for the original diversion are more important than the differences in the two types of ostomies. In a small study of patients with severe underlying illness, advanced age (mean age of 72 years), or widespread malignancy, the closure rate was only 38%.[9] By contrast, in a randomized, multicenter study comparing temporary loop ileostomy with loop colostomy in patients with fewer comorbid conditions and lower mean age (64 years), the closure rate was higher (80%).[6] In this series, there was no significant difference in the closure rates between the types of ostomies.

### New developments

Laparoscopic or minimal access surgery has added a new dimension to the field of colon and rectal surgery. The ability to create a diverting ostomy using laparoscopic techniques has been described by several authors.[19–23] The reduction in the morbidity, mortality, time to return of bowel function, and total length of stay has encouraged further use of laparoscopic intestinal stoma construction. The differences between laparoscopic loop ileostomy and laparoscopic loop colostomy have not been studied, but may reflect trends noted during laparotomy procedures for ostomy creation.

## CONCLUSIONS

Improvements in enterostomal therapy have enhanced satisfaction of patients with both loop ileostomy and transverse loop colostomy. There are similar morbidity and mortality rates for construction and reversal of either form of ostomy. Both types of ostomy provide excellent fecal diversion and protection of distal anastamosis. The development of laparoscopic surgery has changed algorithms for fecal diversion because of the lower morbidity and mortality of this technique compared to laparotomy. However, the lower appliance leak rate, less odor, quicker return of bowel function, and lower prolapse rate all contribute to the superiority of diverting loop ileostomy as compared to colostomy, whether performed by laparoscopy or laparotomy.

## REFERENCES

1    Lahey FH. Surgical intervention in ulcerative colitis. *Ann Surg* 1951;**133**:726

2    Bierman HJ, Tocker AM, Tucker LR. Statistical survey of problems in patients with colostomy or ileostomy. *Am J Surg* 1966;**112**:647–650

3    Schuster MM. Open remarks on artificial openings. *N Engl J Med* 1972;**286**: 891–892

4    Pearl RK, Prasad L, Orsay CP, Abcarian H, Tan AB, Melzl MT. Early local complications from intestinal stomas. *Arch Surg* 1985;**120**:1145–1147

5    Williams NS, Nasmyth DG, Jones D, Smith AH. De-functioning stomas: a prospective controlled trial comparing loop ileostomy with loop transverse colostomy. *Br J Surg* 1986;**73**:566–570

6    Gooszen AW, Geelkerken RH, Hermans J, Lagaay MB, Gooszen HG. Temporary decompression after colorectal surgery: randomized comparison of loop ileostomy and loop colostomy. *Br J Surg* 1998;**85**:76–79

7    Khoury GA, Lewis MCA, Meleagros L, Lewis AAM. Colostomy or ileostomy after colorectal anastomosis?: a randomised trial. *Ann R Coll Surg Engl* 1987;**69**:5–7

8 Chen F, Stuart M. The morbidity of defunctioning stomata. *Aust NZ J Surg* 1996;**66**: 218–221

9 Rutegard J, Dahlgren S. Transverse colostomy or loop ileostomy as diverting stoma in colorectal surgery. *Acta Chir Scand* 1987;**153**:229–232

10 Winslet MC, Barsoum G, Pringle W *et al.* Loop ileostomy after ileal pouch–anal anastamosis – is it necessary? *Dis Colon Rectum* 1991;**34**:267–270

11 Finegold SM, Sutter VL, Boyle JD, Shimada K. The normal flora of ileostomy and transverse colostomy effluents. *J Infect Dis* 1970;**122**:376–381

12 Khoo RE, Cohen MM, Chapman GM, Jenken DA, Langevin JM. Loop ileostomy for temporary fecal diversion. *Am J Surg* 1994;**167**:519–522

13 Hill GL. *Ileostomy: Surgery, Physiology and Management.* Grune and Stratton, New York, 1976

14 Christl SU, Scheppach W. Metabolic consequences of total colectomy. *Scand J Gastroenterol Suppl* 1997;**222**:20–24

15 Feinberg SM, McLeod RS, Cohen Z. Complications of loop ileostomy. *Am J Surg* 1987;**153**:102–107

16 Salum M, Lam D, Wexner SD, *et al.* Does bioresorbable membrane of modified sodium hyaluronate and carboxymethylcellulose (Seprafilm®) have possible short term beneficial impact? *Dis Colon Rectum* (in press)

17 Edwards DP, Donaldson DR, Chisholm EM. Closure of transverse loop colostomy and loop ileostomy. *Ann R Coll Surg Engl* 1998;**80**:33–35

18 Khoury DA, Beck DE, Opelka FG, Hicks TC, Timmcke AE, Gathright B. Colostomy closure: Ochsner clinic experience. *Dis Colon Rectum* 1996;**39**:605–609

19 Hollyoak MA, Lumley J, Stitz RW. Laparoscopic stoma formation for faecal diversion. *Br J Surg* 1998;**85**:226–228

20 Lyerly HK, Mault JR. Laparoscopic ileostomy and colostomy. *Ann Surg* 1994;**219**: 317–322

21 Khoo REH, Montrey J, Cohen MM. Laparoscopic loop ileostomy for temporary fecal diversion. *Dis Colon Rectum* 1993;**36**:966–968

22 Ludwig KA, Milsom JW, Garcia-Ruiz A, Fazio VW. Laparoscopic techniques for fecal diversion. *Dis Colon Rectum* 1996;**39**:285–288

23 Oliveira L, Reissman P, Nogueras J, Wexner SD. Laparoscopic creation of stomas. *Surg Endosc* 1997;**11**:19–23

# 3 Does closure of the wound after excision of a pilonidal sinus improve the result?

*Asha Senapati*

## INTRODUCTION

Many procedures have been described for the management of symptomatic pilonidal sinus, none of which – judged by the yardsticks of primary healing and recurrence of disease – are perfect. Although simple shaving and removal of hair may control symptoms without operation,[1] surgery is often required when chronic infection supervenes. Allen-Mersh, is his review article of 1990, describes outcomes after treatment by a number of methods;[2] these results are summarized in Table 3.1.

A prime requirement of any surgical treatment is the avoidance of major morbidity. In the case of pilonidal disease, the most problematic complication is a persistently unhealed midline wound (Fig. 3.1) most commonly seen after laying open (or excision) of the primary disease or after a failed attempt at primary closure after a wide excision. The exact frequency of this complication is difficult to determine from the literature because many reports detail disease recurrence rather than healing failure.[3–5] However, clinicians who manage this condition regularly are familiar with this vexing situation. Such wounds are often painful, prevent return to normal activity (particularly gainful employment), and usually demand regular nursing and medical attention. These wounds may never heal.

Primarily healing of wounds is probably more satisfactory when wounds are sutured rather than being left to heal by secondary intention, but comparison between methods must take into account failure of healing after primary closure as well as long-term recurrence.

Surgical procedures that keep the main wound away from the midline are said to be more likely to succeed. Karydakis[6] described a technique of asymmetric closure with excellent results. Mann & Springall[7] have also described an asymmetric excision and primary closure with good results but with the use of general anesthesia and a

**Table 3.1** Comparison of the results of different techniques for the treatment of pilonidal sinus disease[2]

| Method | Failure (%) | Recurrence (%) | Series reference No. |
|---|---|---|---|
| Simple laying open | 0–43 | | 2 |
| Wide excision with marsupialization | 1–36 | | 2 |
| Primary midline closure | 0–30 | 0–26 | 2 |
| Asymmetric open wound (Bascom's) | 0.5 | 9.6 | 19 |
| Asymmetric closure (Karydakis) | 3–20 | 0–4 | 7, 14–17 |
| Skin flaps | 0–20 | 0–10 | 22–25, 27, 28 |

**Fig 3.1** Unhealed midline wound in natal cleft: failure of healing after excision of pilonidal sinus.

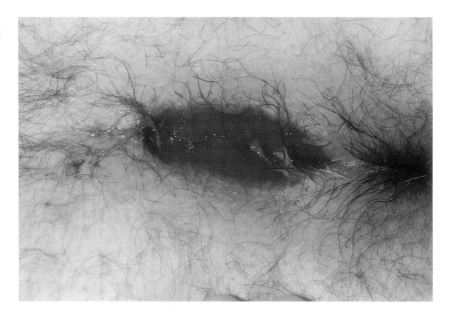

mean hospital stay of 16 days. Bascom's technique,[8,9] an ambulatory procedure undertaken with local anesthesia, which similarly places the main wound away from the midline, also gives good results, but with the disadvantage of an open wound.

In today's financial climate, ambulatory treatments that offer rapid return to full activity, perhaps using local anesthesia, will be preferred to more complex procedures, so long as they are shown to be effective in managing the disease by avoiding long-term unhealed wounds. Such objectives are in keeping with the current requirement to reduce the duration of inpatient hospital stay and treatment costs.

## ETIOLOGY

The etiology of pilonidal sinus is poorly understood. The congenital theory is largely discounted;[2,10] pilonidal sinus is thought to be acquired. Bascom's theory is that pits form under the influence of the gravitational pull on the postanal skin,[11] as a result of the repeated rubbing action of the buttocks. It may be that the operations described fail to remove the precipitating factors and this may account for the high recurrence rate seen. Pilonidal pits are known to occur in skin that has been moved to the midline from elsewhere.[1] Furthermore, missed pits may be a cause for persistent disease; surgeons must make every effort to identify and excise all disease existing at the time of surgery. The potential exists for adhesions to form between the postanal skin and the postsacral fascia, which may account for some recurrent disease after any form of surgical treatment. The uncertainty in the etiology makes this disease difficult to treat. It is apparent that patients outgrow the tendency to symptomatic pilonidal sinus disease, as it is seldom seen over the age of 40 years;[4] this may result from changes in the nature of the hair or postanal skin. It is logical that surgical treatment for this condition should minimize anatomic disruption of the region until this time is reached.

## TREATMENT

Several treatments have been described. This article addresses the issue of wound closure and so nonoperative forms of treatment will not be discussed. They are usually temporizing measures with a poor long-term result. Surgery is usually required for definitive treatment.

Surgical treatments can be divided into those in which the wound is left open and those in which the wound is closed. In addition, operations can be midline or asymmetric.

*Midline operations*
1   Simple laying open.
2   Wide excision with marsupialization.
3   Wide excision with primary midline closure.

*Asymmetric operations with wounds away from midline*
1   Karydakis' operation – asymmetric primary closure.
2   Bascom's procedure – asymmetric wound left open.
3   Bascom's cleft closure – asymmetric primary closure.
4   Rotational flaps.

One of the drawbacks of published research on the results of the different techniques is the very small numbers in several series. Allen-Mersh[2] published a comprehensive review of the literature in which he provided a summary of all the published data (see Table 3.1).

## Midline operations

### Simple laying open
With this technique, the pilonidal tracts are simply laid open, often under local anesthetic, and allowed to heal by secondary intention. The wounds require regular dressings. The average time to healing is 43 days, although there are wide variations between reports.

### Wide excision with marsupialization
This method of treatment is based on the premise that pilonidal sinus disease cannot be treated unless all the fibrous and granulation tissue is excised. This premise is no longer universally accepted. In procedures such as Bascom's operation, where the tracts are not excised, the wounds heal well. Wide excision therefore cannot be justified. Average healing time is 73 days, which can be reduced if the edges of the wound are attached to the presacral fascia. Nonhealing of the wound does occur, but it is difficult to extract from the published literature the true incidence of this complication.

### Wide excision with primary midline closure
This method has the potential advantage of avoiding a wound, thus providing greater patient comfort and return to work. Failure of this method will convert the situation into that of the wide excision and marsupialization technique, with all its disadvantages. Primary healing is achieved in the majority, but in some there is failure of healing, often indefinitely. Good results are more likely in the hands of enthusiasts. The number of people with wounds unhealed at 2 months after primary closure is similar to that of those with wounds unhealed after laying open.[12] The other disadvantages of primary closure are that a general anesthetic and inpatient stay are usually required.

## Asymmetric operations

### Karydakis operation

Karydakis[6,13] described a technique of asymmetric natal cleft wound closure (Fig. 3.2). An eccentric, elliptical excision is made with mobilization of a flap from the medial side of the wound. All sinus tracts are excised completely down to the sacral periosteum. The mobilized flap is sutured to the sacrococcygeal fascia and the wound is closed. The results of this operation have been reported in 7471 patients;[6] it

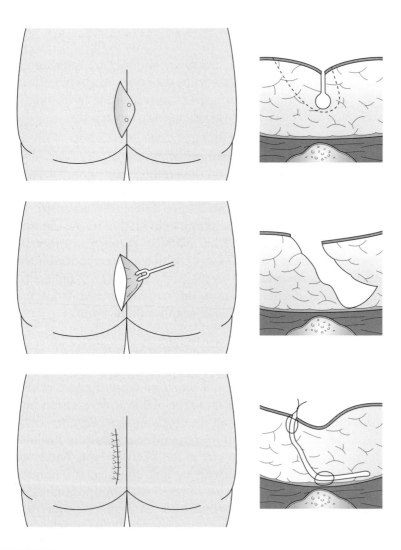

**Fig 3.2** Karydakis technique for pilonidal sinus.

was performed under general anesthesia, with a mean hospital stay of 3 days. These wounds healed well, with a recurrence rate of <1%, results that have been mirrored by others. Patel *et al.*[14] using the Karydakis method, have avoided the situation of an unhealed midline wound, albeit with an inpatient stay of 5 days. Recurrence was not reported but follow up was not complete. Anyanwu *et al.*[15] treated 28 patients by this technique and reported no recurrence after a median follow up of 3 years. Primary healing occurred in 88% of cases and all wounds eventually healed. Patients stayed in hospital an average of 4 days. Kitchen[16] noted a 4% recurrence and a slow healing rate of 3%. Mann & Springall[7] have also described an asymmetric excision and primary closure with good results; they also used general anesthesia, but reported a mean hospital stay of 16 days.

### Bascom's operation

Bascom's technique[8,9,11] is an out patient procedure undertaken under local anesthesia, which similarly places the main wound away from the midline (Fig. 3.3). Midline pits are excised, removing a minimal amount of tissue (equivalent to a grain of rice) in each case. Care is taken to identify all pits by stretching the post-anal skin caudally; these wounds extend into the 'abscess' cavity, which is then drained laterally to the most convenient side of the midline via a parallel incision at a distance of some 2–3 cm. The abscess cavity is curetted, thereby removing all infected granulation tissue and hair. A fibrous and fatty flap (consisting of the lateral wall of the abscess cavity opposite to the lateral drainage incision) is lifted, deep to the midline pits, thus releasing them from the postsacral fascia. This flap is

**Fig 3.3** Bascom's technique for pilonidal sinus.

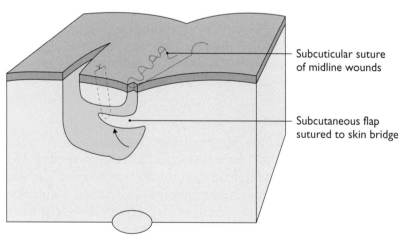

Subcuticular suture of midline wounds

Subcutaneous flap sutured to skin bridge

sutured to the bridge of skin between the midline pits and the lateral drainage wound and the midline wounds are closed with a subcuticular, nonabsorbable suture; 4.0 Prolene on a curved, cutting needle is our preferred material. Hemostasis is then secured using monopolar diathermy.[17]

The lateral drainage wound is neither sutured nor packed and a light dressing is applied to absorb postoperative discharge. All sutures are removed after 1 week and patients are reviewed at weekly intervals until all wounds are healed. Patients are self-caring with no need for attention by a nurse.

It is rare for these wounds not to heal. We have found an average time to healing of 4 weeks. Bascom reports an 8% recurrence rate,[9] which is similar to that for our series (9.6%)[18] and that for Mosquera & Quayle (7.3%).[19]

### Bascom's cleft closure operation

A similar procedure to the Karydakis operation was described by Bascom (Fig. 3.4),[11,20] originally for closing the unhealed midline wound (see below). A flap of skin is raised from the least damaged side of the cleft. The underlying sinuses and abscess cavity are curetted and laid open but are not excised. No fat or muscle is mobilized and the wound lies well outside the sacrococcygeal fascia. The exposed fat is sutured together, thus obliterating the depth of the natal cleft, and the flap of skin is sutured to the opposite side asymmetrically, having excised sufficient tissue to allow this to lie without tension. This operation is far less extensive than the Karydakis operation, and may be done under local anesthesia as an outpatient procedure. Wounds usually heal primarily, but if part of the wound breaks down (often the lower part), it heals rapidly. There are no published results of this cleft closure technique but, to date, 31 patients have been treated for primary and recurrent pilonidal sinus at this institution. All patients' wounds healed, although only 39% did so primarily. There have been no recurrences to date.

### Rotational flaps

Techniques which obliterate the natal cleft are successful in treating chronic pilonidal sinus disease (Fig. 3.5). Tekin[21] treated 162 patients using a rhomboid Limberg flap: the average hospital stay was 4 days; 7% of wounds did not heal primarily but all healed eventually, although 2% of cases recurred. Azab *et al.*[22] reported the results of 30 rhomboid flaps, with 96% primary healing and no recurrences.

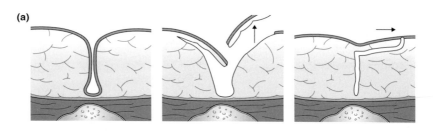

(a)

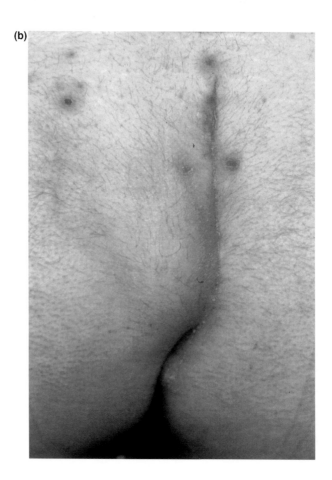

(b)

**Fig 3.4** Bascom's cleft closure technique for the unhealed midline wound and primary pilonidal sinus.

Bozkurt & Tezel[23] and Jimenez *et al.*[24] have had similar results and no recurrences. Z-plasty has also been used successfully.[25]

Mansoory & Dickson[26] treated 120 patients with no wound disruptions and only two recurrences. Other reports have a high failure rate.[27] A comparison of Z-plasty with wide excision and marsupialization found the former to be superior.[28]

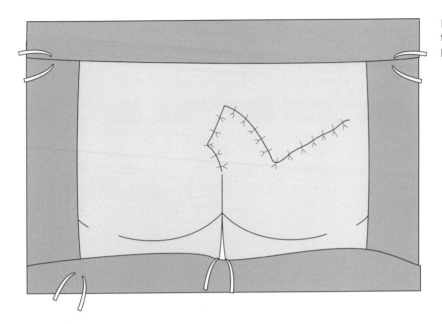

**Fig 3.5** Rhomboid flap for the treatment of pilonidal sinus.

These operations, however, require major surgery and are cosmetically disfiguring. They may be viewed as a 'sledgehammer to crack a nut' and as lesser operations are equally successful, they are probably preferable.

## The unhealed midline wound

It would not be appropriate to discuss wound closure for pilonidal sinus disease without specific reference to unhealed midline wounds, which are almost entirely iatrogenic. Unhealed midline wounds mostly result from the failure of the wounds of excisional surgery for pilonidal sinus disease to heal. These wounds are best avoided altogether by the techniques described above, but patients unfortunate enough to have such wounds clearly need treatment.

Conventionally, such wounds have been treated with regular dressings, ranging from simple gauze to silastic foam, and depilation. Surgical treatment with primary closure usually fails. Cleft closure, as described above, has been advocated by Bascom for this condition.[21,29] In the Portsmouth colorectal unit, we have undertaken 18 of these procedures for unhealed midline wounds: all wounds eventually healed, with 37% healing primarily; there have been no recurrences of the problem. We believe that surgical correction by this technique should be the first line of management of these wounds and that prolonged periods of wound dressing is an inappropriate use of resources.

## CONCLUSIONS

The primary aim of treatment in pilonidal sinus disease is to eradicate sepsis and allow wound healing with minimal morbidity and recurrence. The disease is more often troublesome than dangerous. There is a risk that with certain treatments the consequences of failed treatment will be worse than the disease itself. In a condition that is likely to be self-limiting, use of such treatments is not justified. Leaving widely excised midline wounds to heal by secondary intention is not logical. Laying open has good results but with a failure rate no different to primary closure. Although primary midline closure is usually successful, it fails to heal in a sufficiently large number of patients, so one has to look seriously at the options. Laterally placed wounds fare better as far as healing is concerned. Bascom's operation has excellent results and is quick and simple to perform, with minimal morbidity. It does, however, leave an open wound for a few weeks. Karydakis' operation also has good results, but is a more major operation and is more difficult to perform. Bascom's cleft closure allows primary closure in a laterally placed wound, although this too does not heal primarily in the majority of cases. It is, however, easier to perform than the Karydakis method and can be done under local anesthetic as an outpatient procedure.

The true advantages and benefits of the different techniques can only be compared in the context of randomized trials, which are scarce in the treatment of this disease. Certainly, with more innovative approaches becoming available, the time is ripe for such comparisons. Prolonged time away from work due to unhealed wounds is avoidable: when wounds do not heal, simple surgical techniques can be used to overcome the problem.

## REFERENCES

1   Armstrong JH, Barcia PJ. Pilonidal sinus disease. The conservative approach. *Arch Surg* 1994;**129**:914–917

2   Allen-Mersh TG. Pilonidal sinus: finding the right track for treatment. Review (141 refs). *Br J Surg* 1990;**77**:123–132

3   Bissett IP, Isbister WH. The management of patients with pilonidal disease – a comparative study. *Aust NZ J Surg* 1987;**57**:939–942

4    Clothier PR, Haywood IR. The natural history of the post anal (pilonidal) sinus. *Ann R Coll Surg Engl* 1984;**66**:201–203

5    McLaren CA. Partial closure and other techniques in pilonidal surgery: an assessment of 157 cases. *Br J Surg* 1984;**71**:561–562

6    Karydakis GE. Easy and successful treatment of pilonidal sinus after explanation of its causative process. *Aust NZ J Surg* 1992;**62**:385–389

7    Mann CV, Springall R. 'D' excision for sacrococcygeal pilonidal sinus disease. *J R Soc Med* 1987;**80**:292–295

8    Bascom J. Pilondial disease: long-term results of follicle removal. *Dis Colon Rectum* 1983;**26**:800–807

9    Bascom J. Pilonidal disease: origin from follicles of hairs and results of follicle removal as treatment. *Surgery* 1980;**87**:567–572

10   Brearley R. Pilonidal sinus. A new theory of origin. *Br J Surg* 1955;**43**:62–68

11   Bascom J. Pilonidal sinus. *Current Therapy in Colon and Rectal Surgery*. B C Decker, New York, 1990, p. 329

12   Rainsbury RM, Southam JA. Radical surgery for pilonidal sinus. *Ann R Coll Surg Engl* 1982;**64**:339–341

13   Karydakis GE. New approach to the problem of pilonidal sinus. *Lancet* 1973; **2**:1414–1415

14   Patel H, Lee M, Bloom I, Allen-Mersh TG. Prolonged delay in healing after surgical treatment of pilonidal sinus is avoidable. *Colorectal Dis* 1999; **1**:107–110

15   Anyanwu AC, Hossain S, Williams A, Montgomery AC. Karydakis operation for sacrococcygeal pilonidal sinus disease: experience in a district general hospital. *Ann R Coll Surg Engl* 1998;**80**:197–199

16   Kitchen PR. Pilonidal sinus: experience with the Karydakis flap [see comments]. *Br J Surg* 1996;**83**:1452–1455

17   Senapati A. Pilonidal sinus. *Postgrad Surg* 1996;**6**:19–24

18   Senapati A, Cripps NPJ, Thompson MR. Bascom's operation in the day surgical management of symptomatic pilonidal sinus. *Br J Surg* 2000: in press

19   Mosquera DA, Quayle JB. Bascom's operation for pilonidal sinus. *J R Soc Med* 1995;**88**:45P–46P

20   Bascom JU. Pilonidal sinus. *Curr Pract Surg* 1994;**6**:175–180

21   Tekin A. Pilonidal sinus: experience with the Limberg flap. *Colorectal Dis* 1999;**1**:29–33

22   Azab AS, Kamal MS, Saad RA, Abou al Atta KA, Ali NA. Radical cure of pilonidal sinus by a transposition rhomboid flap. *Br J Surg* 1984;**71**:154–155

23   Bozkurt MK, Tezel E. Management of pilonidal sinus with the Limberg flap. *Dis Colon Rectum* 1998;**41**:775–777

24   Jimenez RC, Alcalde M, Martin F, Pulido A, Rico P. Treatment of pilonidal sinus by excision and rhomboid flap. *Int J Colorectal Dis* 1990;**5**:200–202

25   Toubanakis G. Treatment of pilonidal sinus disease with the Z-plasty procedure (modified). *Am Surg* 1986;**52**:611–612

26   Mansoory A, Dickson D. Z-plasty for treatment of disease of the pilonidal sinus. *Surg Gynecol Obstet* 1982;**155**:409–411

27   Morrison PD. Is Z-plasty closure reasonable in pilonidal disease? *Ir J Med Sci* 1985;**154**:110–112

28   Hodgson WJ, Greenstein RJ. A comparative study between Z-plasty and incision and drainage or excision with marsupialization for pilonidal sinuses. *Surg Gynecol Obstet* 1981;**153**:842–844

29   Bascom JU. Repeat pilonidal operations. *Am J Surg* 1987;**154**:118–122

# 4 Can anal fissures be treated without surgery?

*Paul B Boulos and James Pitt*

## INTRODUCTION

An idiopathic anal fissure is a common condition which constitutes 13% of referrals to a coloproctology clinic.[1] An anal fissure occurs equally in both sexes, usually in young adults, and is rare in the elderly. A fissure is a linear tear in the squamous lining of the lower half of the anal canal, between the anal verge and the dentate line; it is more commonly seen in both genders in the posterior midline. Although posterior fissures are more common than are anterior ones, anterior midline fissures are more common in females.[2] The breach in the mucosa is initially superficial, but may extend to the underlying internal anal sphincter if it remains unhealed. The fissure is defined as chronic when it is symptomatic for more than 3 months or when it shows secondary changes, consisting of undermined rolled edges with visible pale internal sphincter fibers at its base, a hypertrophied anal papilla at its proximal end, and a skin tag known as a sentinel pile at its distal edge.[1] The presenting symptoms are usually pain on defecation, bleeding and pruritus and the classical signs are tenderness at the site of the fissure on digital palpation of the anal verge and sphincter spasm which prohibits digital insertion and full rectal examination. Based upon these signs, symptoms, and physical findings, the diagnosis of fissure can be secured without a digital rectal examination or anoscopy.

## TREATMENT RATIONALE

Although several factors have been implicated in the pathogenesis of this condition, the precise etiology remains elusive. Therapy has, therefore, evolved around our understanding of the physiologic abnormality, which is increased internal anal sphincter activity, resulting in a high anal canal pressure that compromises the mucosal blood flow in the posterior commissure, where the blood supply is already deficient,[3] delaying healing of the fissure.[4] Laser Doppler studies have demonstrated poor blood flow in patients with a chronic fissure which is improved following sphincterotomy.[5] It is not known whether the high pressures cause the fissure or vice versa. Different therapeutic modalities have aimed at reducing the anal canal pressure, which cures this condition, although at the expense of disturbing the sphincter mechanism. The efficacy of treatment is measured therefore by its cure rate and its effect on continence.

## SURGICAL TREATMENT

### Manual dilatation

Recamier,[6] as early as 1838, recommended anal dilatation as a treatment for anal fissure. The technique is simple and pain relief is immediate; however, recurrence rates as high as 57% and minor anal incontinence in up to 28% of patients have been reported (Table 4.1). These results are unfavorable compared with posterior and lateral internal sphincterotomy, as has been confirmed in controlled studies.[9,13] However, excellent outcome following manual dilatation in more than one series challenges the supremacy of lateral anal sphincterotomy.[12,14] In a prospective trial of 111 patients randomized between manual dilatation and subcutaneous sphincterotomy, the recurrence and incontinence rates were similar at 5% or less.[15] However, there is an undoubted risk of damage to both the internal

**Table 4.1** Results and complications of manual dilatation of the anus

| Study | Number | Minor anal incontinence* (%) | Major anal incontinence (%) | Recurrence/ nonhealing (%) |
|---|---|---|---|---|
| Watts et al.[7] | 99 | 28 | 2 | 16 |
| MacIntyre & Balfour[8] | 55 | 22 | 3.6 | — |
| Saad & Omer[9] | 37 | 22 | 2.8 | 8.1 |
| MacDonald et al.[10] | 46 | 20 | 4 | 57 |
| Nielsen et al.[11] | 32 | 13 | 0 | 12 |
| Isbister & Prasad[12] | 104 | 0 | 0 | 4.8 |

*Fecal soiling and flatus incontinence.

and external anal sphincters caused by manual dilatation, which has been documented on endoanal ultrasonography.[11,16]

Sohn and his colleagues[17] have successfully treated patients without disturbance of continence by gradual and controlled dilatation, using a Park's anal retractor or hydrostatic balloon. This technique has never gained popularity.

## Posterior anal sphincterotomy

Incising the exposed internal sphincter at the base of the fissure was initially suggested in 1833 by Dupuytren[18] and was reintroduced by Eisenhammer in 1951.[19] In 1930, Gabriel[20] advocated excision of the fissure incorporating the internal sphincter. This method of treatment cures 95% of fissures, but the major drawback with posterior sphincterotomy with or without fissurectomy is related to the wound, which takes at least 6 weeks to heal, compared with 3 weeks after lateral sphincterotomy.[13,21] The healed wound leaves a cicatricial groove in the midline (keyhole deformity) that has been incriminated in the high incontinence rates reported in several series (Table 4.2). Bode and colleagues[23] treated 121 patients with a low complication and recurrence rate and without any loss of continence. The authors attributed this success to careful technique in limiting the incision to

**Table 4.2** Results and complications of posterior internal anal sphincterotomy

| Study | Number | Minor anal incontinence*/ mucus leak (%) | Major anal incontinence (%) | Recurrence (%) |
|---|---|---|---|---|
| Hawley[13] | 32 | 6.7 | 0 | 6.7 |
| Abcarian[21] | 150 | 5 | 0 | 1.3 |
| Hsu & MacKeigan[22] | 344 | 0.2 | 0 | 13.1 |
| Bode et al.[23] | 121 | 0 | 0 | 1.3 |
| Khubchandani & Reed[24] | 58 | 31 | 5 | — |
| Jost et al.[25] | 113 | 28.4 | 2.2 | 1.8 |
| Saad & Omer[9] | 21 | 9.5 | 0 | 0 |

*Fecal soiling and flatus incontinence.

the superficial fibers of the internal sphincter. However, a posterior sphincterotomy is unavoidable when the fissure is complicated by an intersphincteric abscess or a fistula.[21,25]

## Lateral anal sphincterotomy

Parks[26] in 1967 popularized the open technique of lateral sphincterotomy first introduced by Boyer[27] in 1818. In 1969 Notaras[28] developed the subcutaneous technique. The sphincter is divided at its lateral margin, at 3 or 9 o'clock, away from the fissure, which is left intact. A sentinel pile or a hypertrophied anal papilla is excised only when large and troublesome. The operation provides immediate symptomatic improvement and the fissure heals within 3 weeks in about 95% of cases, with minor incontinence in less than 3%, usually due to flatus,[2,29,30] which recovers in most instances (Table 4.3). The therapeutic advantage of lateral sphincterotomy over posterior sphincterotomy and manual dilatation has been validated in comparative studies.[2,10,21,25] The clinical outcome and the adequacy of

**Table 4.3** Results and complications of lateral internal sphincterotomy

| Study | Number | Minor anal incontinence* (%) | Major anal incontinence (%) | Recurrence/ nonhealing (%) |
|---|---|---|---|---|
| Bailey et al.[29] | 418 | 2.2 | 0.2 | 0.7 |
| Boulos & Araujo[30] | 14 | 21 | 0 | 0 |
| Vafai & Mann[31] | 697 | 1 | 0 | 5.5 |
| Lewis et al.[32] | 247 | 6.9 | 0 | 5.3 |
| Khubchandani & Reed[24] | 292 | 38 | 6 | 2.3 |
| Kortbeek et al.[33] | 58 | 0 | 0 | 3.4 |
| Pernikoff et al.[34] | 290 | 8 | 0.5 | 2.9 |
| Oh et al.[2] | 1391 | 15 | 0 | 1.3 |
| Garcia-Aguilar et al.[35] | 549 | 37.8 | 8.2 | 11.1 |
| Littlejohn & Newstead[36] | 352 | 1.75 | 0 | 1.75 |

*Fecal soiling and flatus incontinence.

sphincterotomy, as measured by reduction in resting anal canal pressure after either open or subcutaneous sphincterotomy, are similar.[31–33]

Lateral sphincterotomy has been performed safely and effectively under local anesthesia, although inadequate division of the sphincter, and hence recurrence, may pose a problem.[37] Dexterity in technique may not be as simple in the conscious patient and the procedure is more demanding. Abcarian[21] performed 150 procedures using local anesthesia with a 1.3% recurrence; none of the patients had a disturbance of continence.

The long-term follow up has aroused concern: in one report, 8% of patients were incontinent of flatus and had fecal soiling over 10 years,[34] and minor incontinence was even higher in other reports.[24,35] These disturbing observations were related to the extent of sphincter division. Endosonography has shown that in some patients, the defect in the sphincter involved its full length, particularly in women who, anatomically, have a shorter anal canal.[38] A standard landmark for the proximal limit of sphincter division has been the dentate line and this should be at an even lower level in females. Sphincterotomy restricted to the length of the fissure has been reported to reduce incontinence to 1.4% at long-term follow up without jeopardizing the cure rate.[36]

## Anal advancement flap

The V–Y advancement technique was employed by Dieffenbach in 1848 for the correction of anal strictures[39] and has been applied to cover the raw surface in chronic anal fissures. This treatment is as favorable as lateral sphincterotomy and does not interfere with the sphincter mechanism.[22,40] In Leong & Seow-Choen randomized 20 patients to lateral sphincterotomy and 20 patients to an advancement flap; all fissures healed except those in three patients in the flap group with a median length of hospital stay of 2 days. No patient was incontinent and patient satisfaction with surgery was similar for the two groups.[40]

Flaps were particularly indicated to treat recurrent anal fissures after adequate sphincterotomy and in patients with low resting pressures, such as elderly patients and multiparous and postpartum women; 9% of postpartum women develop anal fissures unrelated to the mode of delivery.[41] Nyam *et al.* reported on 21 patients (six men and 15 women) with low resting and maximum squeeze pressures, of whom nine had had a previous lateral sphincterotomy and 15 showed defects in the anal sphincters on endoanal ultrasonography. All underwent flap repair with a median hospital stay of 3 (range 2–8) days. All flaps healed with preservation of sensation. Continence was maintained in all patients. At a median follow up of 18 (range 6–28) months all fissures healed.[42]

# NONSURGICAL TREATMENT

## Conservative management

In a study of 393 patients treated with cautery, suppositories, and sitz baths, although 44% of patients' wounds healed in the short term, 27% of this group developed recurrent anal fissures over a 5-year follow-up period.[43] The acute episode of anal fissure resolved in 87% of patients treated with warm sitz baths and unprocessed bran. When the unprocessed bran was taken daily, the recurrence rates were significantly lower among patients who continued to take 15 g bran (16%) compared with those taking 7.5 g bran (60%) or no added fiber (68%).[44] Gough & Lewis[45] reported that 1 month after treatment, fissures healed in 43.6% of patients using 2% lidocaine gel alone and in 41.9% of patients who also used an anal dilator. The addition of topical agents does not appear to improve healing and is likely to cause skin allergy.[46] Although the application of anesthetic agents or steroids may be beneficial in relieving acute symptoms, the same effect is achieved faster with unprocessed bran. Lock & Thomson[1] reported that 54% of their patients treated by local anesthetic agents and bulk laxatives were relieved of their symptoms, but long-term follow up indicated that healing was maintained in only half of these patients. Factors that were found to be associated with a poor long-term outcome following conservative treatment and the need for surgery were the presence of a skin tag and a fibrous polyp. The use of anal dilators as part of the conservative treatment is distasteful and painful and has been shown to be of no added benefit to the use of stool softeners and topical anesthetics alone.[45,47]

Although these different medications are readily available and may have a role in the short term for symptomatic relief, their effect is not immediate and the cure, except for acute fissures, is unpredictable.

## Chemical sphincterotomy

This term appropriately refers to pharmacologic manipulation of anal sphincter tone as an alternate modality. Chemical sphincterotomy appears to be as to effective as lateral sphincterotomy in reducing anal canal pressure, which facilitates healing of fissures without permanently disrupting normal sphincter function. This option has been made possible with a broader understanding of the physiologic mechanism controlling smooth muscle contraction.

Internal anal sphincter smooth muscle relaxation is mediated by the stimulation of nitric oxide releasing nonadrenergic, noncholinergic enteric neurons. It is also effected by stimulation of parasympathetic muscarinic receptors, sympathetic β-adrenergic receptors or by direct inhibition of calcium entry into the cell. The muscle contraction is dependent on an increase in cytoplasmic calcium and is also enhanced by sympathetic α-adrenergic stimulation.[48]

Currently, the most commonly used pharmacologic agent in the treatment of fissures is topical glyceryl trinitrate (GTN). Other agents that exhibit a similar effect through inhibition of calcium channels, muscarinic-receptor stimulation, α-adrenergic inhibition, or β-adrenergic stimulation are also demonstrating a therapeutic potential.

## Nitric oxide donors

Nitric oxide is the sole neurotransmitter that mediates neurogenic relaxation of the human internal anal sphincter, although other neurotransmitters may also play a part.[49] Exogenous sources of nitric oxide, such as sodium nitroprusside, have been shown to mimic this effect *in vitro*.[49] Glyceryl trinitrate is an organic nitrate that binds to protein receptors, releasing nitric oxide and thus acting as a nitric oxide donor. It is available as an ointment for topical administration, and isosorbide dinitrate (ISDN) can be used similarly.[50]

Nitric oxide donors promote healing of anal fissures by increasing local blood flow, by reducing the intra-anal pressure, and by vasodilatation of the vessels supplying the anal musculature. Following successful treatment of fissures with topical GTN or ISDN, the blood flow in the anal mucosa has been shown, using laser Doppler flowmetry, to increase,[50,51] although in one study it remained unaltered.[52]

Glyceryl trinitrate ointment in a 0.2% concentration, applied twice daily for 6 weeks, results in a reduction in anal pressure of 14–44%, and healing rates of 41–86% after variable periods[50–67] (Table 4.4). In randomized controlled trials, 46–70% healing was achieved in the GTN-treated groups compared with 8–32% in the control groups.[51,52,63]

**Table 4.4** Results and complications of use of glyceryl trinitrate (GTN) ointment

| Study | Number | Concentration of GTN (%) | Anal pressure reduction (%) | Healing rate at 6 weeks (%) | Headache (%) |
|---|---|---|---|---|---|
| Loder et al.[53] | 20 | 0.2 | 27 | — | 10 |
| Gorfine[54] | 14 | 0.3 | — | 43 | 29 |
| Gorfine[55] | 3 | 0.5 | — | 0 | 35 |
| Schouten et al.[50] | 16 | 1[a] | — | 56 | 100 |
| Lund et al.[56] | 2 | 0.4 | — | — | 100 |
|  | 21 | 0.2 | 41 | 85.7 | 19 |
| Watson et al.[57] | 19 | 0.2–0.8 | 44.4 | 47 | — |
| Lund & Scholefield[51] | 40 | 0.2 | 33 | 68 | 58 |
| Lund & Scholefield[58] | 39 | 0.2 | 41 | 85.6 | 20 |
| Bacher et al.[59] | 8 | 0.2 | 20 | 62.5 | — |
| Oettle[60] | 12 | [b] | — | 83 | — |
| RCS (Engl)[61] | 295 | 0.2[c] | — | 68 | — |
| Manookian et al.[62] | 21 | 0.2–1[a] | — | 54 | — |
| Carapeti et al.[52] | 23 | 0.2 | — | 70 | 72 |
|  | 23 | 0.2–0.6 | — | 70 | 72 |
| Kennedy et al.[63] | 24 | 0.2 | 14 | 46 | 29 |
| Jonas et al.[64] | 49 | 0.2 | — | 45 | — |
| Hyman & Cataldo[65] | 17 | 0.3 | — | 41 | 88 |
| Brisinda et al.[66] | 25 | 0.2 | — | 60 | 20 |
| Pitt et al.[67] | 45 | 0.2 | — | 49 | 58 |

[a] Isosorbide dinitrate.
[b] Crushed 0.5 mg GTN tablet.
[c] 75% of group.
RCS, Royal College of Surgeons.

The limitation of GTN at higher concentrations is the frequency and severity of headaches, although Gorfine[54] used 0.3% with the same tolerance as with 0.2%. Watson and colleagues[57] reported that 15 of 19 (79%) patients with chronic anal fissures required GTN ointment in a concentration >0.2% to lower the maximum resting pressure by 25%. At 6 weeks, nine patients (47%) had healed, of whom eight required a GTN concentration of >0.3%. Three patients developed tachyphylaxis. Carapeti *et al.*[52] compared 0.2% with 0.2% increasing weekly by 0.1% to a maximum of 0.6% three times daily to counteract tachyphylaxis. After 8 weeks, fissures healed in 67% of patients, with no significant difference between the two treatments; 33% of those healed with 0.2% GTN and 25% of those healed with the escalating dose of GTN recurred. Headaches were reported by 72% of patients. Although doses of up to 0.6% were tolerated because of the gradual increase in dose, this offered only a slight advantage to the speed of healing.

Oettle[60] randomized 24 patients into lateral anal sphincterotomy or GTN treatment using a 0.5 mg tablet of GTN crushed in 10 ml of glycerin lubricating jelly. All patients were healed in the sphincterotomy group and 83% in the GTN group, and there were no adverse effects in either group. He concluded that GTN should be used as the first-line treatment for anal fissure.

Between 56 and 80% of acute fissures can be healed with GTN ointment.[55,62,65] Bacher *et al.*[59] randomized 22 patients with acute fissures into receiving GTN ointment or lidocaine gel; after 1 month, 11 out of 12 fissures healed within 2 weeks with GTN ointment and none with lidocaine gel.

Although there is clearly a therapeutic role for GTN in the treatment of anal fissures, unresolved issues are related to compliance outside clinical trials and the risk of recurrence in the long term. Compliance rates as low as 67% have been reported.[68] Almost all patients treated with GTN ointment develop headaches and nearly 10% of patients abandon treatment for this reason.[61,67,68] Following cessation of treatment with GTN, anal pressures rise to pretreatment levels[69] and therefore patients treated by chemical sphincterotomy may be at risk of recurrent anal fissures. However, while 17–45% of healed fissures recur[67,68] within 36 weeks, they are amenable to further treatment with GTN. In a medium-term follow up (median of 28 months) after successful initial treatment with GTN, 30 of 41 patients (73%) remained symptom-free and of the 11 patients with recurrent symptoms, six responded to a further course of GTN, the fissures of two healed spontaneously, and three required sphincterotomy.[70]

Lysy et al.[71] treated 41 patients with ISDN in a dose of 1.25 mg or 2.5 mg three times daily for 4 weeks. Patients were followed up for an average of 11 months. In 34 (83%) patients the fissure healed within 1 month of treatment. In six (14.6%) patients the fissure did not heal, even after 4 weeks of further treatment, and they underwent lateral sphincterotomy. Six patients relapsed during the follow-up period but responded to another course of treatment. A dose of 2.5 mg of ISDN caused a greater reduction of maximum anal resting pressure than a dose of 1.25 mg and was recommended as the optimal dose.

Schouten et al.[50] treated 34 patients with chronic anal fissure with ISDN, 1 g of 1% ointment applied 3 hourly for 6–12 weeks, with an 88% healing rate. Manometry performed 1 hour after application of ISDN ointment showed a significant reduction of the maximum resting anal pressure. Simultaneous recording of anodermal flow showed a significant increase. During a mean follow-up period of 11 months, relapse of fissure occurred in 2 of 30 patients (7%) at 8 and 10 weeks after discontinuation of therapy.

## Botulinum toxin

*Clostridium botulinum* produces several toxins, of which types A, B, and E have been linked to cases of botulism in humans. Botulinum toxin type A has been found to be of therapeutic value in a number of neurologic and ophthalmologic disorders. The toxin A causes paralysis by rapidly binding to presynaptic cholinergic nerve terminals; it is internalized, inhibiting the release of acetylcholine into the synaptic gap at the neuromuscular junction. A paresis of the injected muscle occurs within hours, which is maximal at 1 week and lasts for up to 3 months. Reinnervation occurs through sprouting of nerve endings within 2 days.[72]

Botulinum toxin is measured in international units (IU), where one unit is the amount of toxin required to kill 50% of a group of mice when injected intraperitoneally ($LD_{50}$ test).[73] There are two commercially available preparations of toxin A – Botox (Allergan Pharmaceuticals, Irvine, CA, USA) and Dysport (Ipsen Ltd, Berkshire, UK).

Jost & Schimrigk[74] first introduced botulinum toxin A in 1993 and successfully treated one patient with a chronic anal fissure; two 1ng doses of toxin diluted to 0.1 ml each containing 2.5 units of Botox, in an insulin syringe were injected with a 27-gauge needle into the external anal sphincter on both sides of the fissure. The pain was relieved by the next day and healing occurred by 12 weeks.

Gui *et al.*[75] claimed to inject the internal sphincter in treating 10 patients with 5 units of Botox on either side and an injection posteriorly. At 2 months, 70% of fissures healed, with a reduction in the resting and squeeze pressures, and one patient developed flatus incontinence.

In various doses of botulinum toxin A, 50–90% of chronic fissures were healed after 6 weeks; up to 12% of patients developed temporary minor fecal incontinence, and 10% of patients had perianal thrombosis secondary to the injection[66,75–84] (Table 4.5).

**Table 4.5** Results and complications of use of botulinum toxin A

| Study | Number | Dose/units | Healing rate (%) | Temporary incontinence (%) | Recurrence (%) | Complications (%) |
|---|---|---|---|---|---|---|
| *Botox** | | | | | | |
| Jost & Schimrigk[76] | 12 | 5 | 83 | 0 | 8 | 0 |
| Gui et al.[75] | 10 | 15 | 70 | 10 | 20 | 10 |
| Jost et al.[77] | 54 | 5 | 78 | 6 | 6 | 11 |
| Jost[78] | 100 | 5 | 82 | 7 | 6 | 0 |
| Espi et al.[79] | 18 | 15 | 81 | 0 | 0 | 0 |
| | 18 | 10 | 65 | 0 | 0 | 0 |
| Maria et al.[80] | 15 | 20 | 73 | 0 | 0 | 0 |
| Brisinda et al.[66] | 25 | 20 | 96 | 0 | 0 | 0 |
| Gonzales et al.[81] | 40 | 15 | 50 | 5 | 0 | 0 |
| Minguez et al.[82] | 23 | 10 | 83 | 0 | 52 | 0 |
| | 27 | 15 | 78 | 0 | 30 | 0 |
| | 19 | 21 | 90 | 0 | 37 | 0 |
| *Dysport* | | | | | | |
| Mason et al.[83] | 5 | Variable | 60 | 0 | 0 | 0 |
| Jost & Schrank[84] | 25 | 20 | 76 | 4 | 0 | 0 |
| | 25 | 40 | 80 | 12 | 0 | 0 |

*2.5 units of Botox is equivalent to 1 ng of pure toxin.

Following injection, there is a reduction in resting pressure and an increase in rectal compliance at 1 week with no change in the squeeze pressure, the anorectal inhibitory reflex, the pudendal nerve terminal motor latency, or electromyography.[73,80] Gui *et al.*[75] however, reported a reduction in squeeze pressure as well.

In a large series of 100 patients treated with 5 units of Botox, 78% of patients were free of pain at 1 week; the fissures of 82% were healed at 3 months, 6% recurred by 6 months, and half of these were cured with further treatment. Interestingly, patients with secondary changes described as large sentinel piles and subfascial infiltration were excluded, although all were classified as chronic because of a 3 month history and all had had at least 2 months of conventional treatment.[78]

Maria *et al.*[80] reported the only randomized controlled trial comparing injections of botulinum toxin A with saline in 30 patients. After 2 months, the fissures of 73% of individuals in the treated group had healed without any recurrences or complications, compared with 13% in the control group. One patient from the control group later treated with botulinum toxin A developed temporary flatus incontinence. There was some disparity in the randomization, in that the control group had more men and was older; nevertheless the result is convincing.

Espi *et al.*[79] injected 20 patients with 5 units of Botox on either side of the fissure and 16 patients with an additional 5 units below the fissure. The healing was 65% and 81%, respectively. Minguez *et al.*[82] compared 10, 15, and 21 units and reported significant reduction in resting and squeeze pressures and higher healing rates without complications using 21 units. Therefore, higher doses of Botox appear to be more effective. Conversely, Jost & Schrank[84] in a series of 50 patients, injected 10 units and 20 units of Dysport adjacent to the fissure margins, and found that the fissures healed in 78% of patients by 3 months. Although there was no significant difference in healing between the two groups, those on the higher dosage showed higher incidence of transient incontinence.

In a controlled trial, 50 patients with chronic anal fissures were randomized to treatment with either 20 units of Botox or 0.2% GTN ointment. After 2 months, 96% of fissures were healed in the Botox group compared with 60% in the GTN group.[66]

Despite the reported success of botulinum toxin A, its use has been limited probably due to patients' aversion to injections and its cost. The optimal dose and method of administration will require validation should this treatment gain wider application.

## Calcium channel antagonists

Calcium channel antagonists inhibit contraction of muscle by preventing calcium influx into the cytoplasm via membrane channels. A placebo-controlled trial using 60 mg diltiazem orally reduced anal resting pressure by 21% compared with 3% in volunteers, but caused some postural dizziness.[85] In the same group of patients, 2% diltiazem gel was used topically, which reduced testing pressure by 28% without adverse effect. Fifteen patients with chronic anal fissure were treated with 2% diltiazem gel, and healing occurred in 67% with no complications.[86]

Sublingual 20 mg nifedipine reduced anal resting pressures by 30% in 10 patients with hemorrhoids or fissures and 10 volunteers.[87] An oral dose of nifedipine retard of 20 mg twice daily was used to treat 15 patients with chronic anal fissure. The initial dose caused a 36% reduction in mean resting pressure and healing was achieved in 60% by 8 weeks.[88] The principal side-effect associated with oral nifedipine was flushing, though this was short-lived.

In a recent prospective randomized double-blind study,[89] 144 patients with acute anal fissures were treated with topical 0.2% nifedipine gel every 12 hours for 3 weeks. The control group, consisting of 142 patients, received topical 1% lidocaine and 1% hydrocortisone gel. Healing was achieved in 95% of the nifedipine-treated patients as opposed to 50% of the controls ($P < 0.01$). The maximum resting pressure decreased by 30% but there was no change in controls. There were no side-effects with nifedipine treatment.

## Cholinergic agonists

A topical gel of the cholinergic agonist, bethanechol, reduced anal resting pressure by 24% in volunteers. In 15 patients with chronic anal fissure treated with 0.1% bethanechol gel, healing occurred in 60% after 8 weeks.[86] This is another promising drug but it has not been evaluated in a controlled trial.

## Alpha-adrenoceptor antagonists and beta-adrenoceptor agonists

In patients with chronic anal fissure, an oral 20 mg dose of the $\alpha_1$-adrenoceptor agonist, indoramin, reduced anal resting pressure by

$36\%^{90}$ and an oral 4 mg dose of the $\beta_2$-adrenoceptor agonist, salbutamol, reduced resting pressure by $23\%$.[91] However, the potential role of these drugs in the treatment of anal fissures has yet to be defined.

## CONCLUSIONS

With several randomized controlled trials as well as many uncontrolled trials supporting the use of both GTN and botulinum toxin A for the treatment of chronic anal fissure, a change in approach in management of chronic anal fissure may be justifiable. Although the cure rate may not seem as high as following surgical treatment, the preservation of continence makes it a more attractive alternative, particularly in certain groups of patients.

There is general acceptance that 0.2% GTN is the optimal therapeutic dose, although a higher dose may accelerate healing and reduce recurrence. GTN causes headaches in almost all patients, especially at the beginning of treatment, and there is some concern about tachyphylaxis. However, there are alternative drugs which are promising. Diltiazem and nifedipine are in the early stages of evaluation and so are many other similar agents, and these may prove to be as effective as, and safer than, GTN.

The dose of botulinum toxin A is less clearly defined: 20 units of Botox has been shown to be superior to lower doses, whereas forty units of Dysport are no more effective than 20 units. There do not seem to be any significant adverse effects with either preparation, although patients might prefer the application of an ointment to an injection. However, the single trial comparing the two treatments showed botulinum toxin A to be superior to GTN ointment. This may be related to higher compliance obtained with botulinum toxin.

Sigmoidoscopy is often impossible in patients with anal fissure because of pain. Five percent of patients with anal fissure have an abnormal finding on rigid sigmoidoscopy.[1] The adoption of nonsurgical treatment does not allow examination under anesthesia routinely performed at the time of surgery. There have been two reports of anorectal carcinoma being initially treated with GTN ointment.[92] Therefore, a careful rectal examination should be the routine once the fissure has healed.

The authors propose that patients should be initially treated with 0.2% GTN or botulinum toxin A. Internal anal sphincterotomy should be reserved for those patients who are not compliant or do not respond to chemical sphincterotomy, with clear warnings of the risk of minor incontinence.

Chemical sphincterotomy is particularly indicated in patients with clinically low anal sphincter tone: namely, elderly patients and women with a past history of difficult childbirth or immediately postpartum. Internal sphincterotomy should be avoided or only considered after careful assessment by endoanal ultrasonography and anal manometry, although an anal advancement flap is the safest option.

# REFERENCES

1    Lock MR, Thomson JPS. Fissure-in-ano: the initial management and prognosis. *Br J Surg* 1977;**64**:355–358

2    Oh C, Divino CM, Steinhagen RM. Anal fissure. 20-year experience. *Dis Colon Rectum* 1995;**38**:378–382

3    Klosterhalfen B, Vogel P, Rixen H, Mittermayer C. Topography of the inferior rectal artery: a possible cause of chronic, primary anal fissure. *Dis Colon Rectum* 1989;**32**:43–52

4    Gibbons CP, Read NW. Anal hypertonia in fissures: cause or effect? *Br J Surg* 1986;**73**:443–445

5    Schouten WR, Briel JW, Auwerda JJA. Relationship between anal pressure and anodermal bloodflow. The vascular pathogenesis of anal fissures. *Dis Colon Rectum* 1994;**37**:664–669

6    Recamier JCA. *Rev Med Fr et Estrang* 1838;**1**:74

7    Watts JM, Bennet RC, Goligher JC. Stretching of anal sphincters in treatment of fissure-in-ano. *Br Med J* 1964;**2**:342–343

8    MacIntyre IMC, Balfour TW. Results of the Lord non-operative treatment for haemorrhoids. *Lancet* 1972;**1**:1094–1095

9    Saad AMA, Omer A. Surgical treatment of chronic fissure-in-ano: a prospective randomised study. *E Afr Med J* 1992;**69**:613–615

10   MacDonald A, Smith A, McNeill AD, Finley IG. Manual dilatation of the anus. *Br J Surg* 1992;**79**:1381–1382

11   Nielsen MB, Rasmussen OO, Pedersen JF, Christiansen J. Risk of sphincter damage and anal incontinence after anal dilatation for fissure-in ano. An endosonographic study. *Dis Colon Rectum* 1993;**36**:677–680

12   Isbister WH, Prasad J. Fissure in ano. *Aust NZ J Surg* 1995;**65**:107–108

13   Hawley PR. The treatment of chronic fissure-in-ano. *Br J Surg* 1969;**56**:915–918

14   Strugnell NA, Cooke SG, Lucarotti ME, Thomson WH. Controlled digital anal dilatation under total neuromuscular blockade for chronic anal fissure: a justifiable procedure. *Br J Surg* 1999;**86**:651–655

15   Weaver RM, Ambrose NS, Alexander-Williams J, Keighley MRB. Manual dilatation of the anus *vs* lateral subcutaneous sphincterotomy in the treatment of chronic fissure in ano. *Dis Colon Rectum* 1987;**30**:420–423

16   Speakman CTM, Burnett SJD, Kamm MA, Bartram CI. Sphincter injury after anal dilatation demonstrated by anal ultrasonography. *Br J Surg* 1991;78:1429–1430

17   Sohn N, Eisenberg MM, Weinstein MA, Lugo RN, Ader J. Precise anorectal dilation. Its role in the therapy of anal fissures. *Dis Colon Rectum* 1992;35:322–327

18   Dupuytren G. *Lecons orales de cliniques chirugicale* 1833;3:284. Germer-Bailliere, Paris.

19   Eisenhammer S. The surgical correction of chronic anal (sphincteric) contracture. *S Afr Med J* 1951;25:486–489

20   Gabriel WB. The treatment of pruritis ani and anal fissure. *Br Med J* 1930;311–312

21   Abcarian H. Surgical correction of chronic anal fissures: results of lateral internal sphincterotomy versus fissurectomy-midline sphincterotomy. *Dis Colon Rectum* 1980;23:31–36

22   Hsu T-C, MacKeigan JM. Surgical treatment of chronic anal fissure. A retrospective study of 1753 cases. *Dis Colon Rectum* 1984;27:475–478

23   Bode WE, Culp CE, Spencer RJ, Beart RW. Fissurectomy with superficial midline sphincterotomy. *Dis Colon Rectum* 1984;27:93–95

24   Khubchandani IT, Reed JF. Sequelae of internal sphincterotomy for chronic fissure in ano. *Br J Surg* 1989;76:431–434

25   Jost WH, Raulf F, Muller-Lobeck H. Anal fissures: results of surgical treatment. *Coloproctology* 1991;13:110–113

26   Parks AG. The management of fissure-in-ano. *Hosp Med* 1967;1:737–738

27   Boyer A. *J Compl Dict Sc Med* (Paris) 1818;2:24

28   Notaras MJ. Lateral subcutaneous sphincterotomy for anal fissure: a new technique. *J R Soc Med* 1969;62:713

29   Bailey RV, Rubin RJ, Salvati EP. Lateral anal sphincterotomy. *Dis Colon Rectum* 1978;21:584–586

30   Boulos PB, Araujo JGC. Adequate internal sphincterotomy for chronic anal fissure: subcutaneous or open technique? *Br J Surg* 1984;71:360–362

31   Vafai M, Mann CV. Closed lateral internal anal sphincterotomy as an office procedure for the treatment of anal fissures. *Coloproctology* 1987;9:49–53

32   Lewis TM, Corman ML, Prager ED, Robertson WG. Long-term results of open and closed sphincterotomy for anal fissure. *Dis Colon Rectum* 1988;31:368–371

33   Kortbeek JB, Langevin JM, Khoo REH, Heine JA. Chronic fissure-in-ano: a randomized study comparing open and subcutaneous lateral sphincterotomy. *Dis Colon Rectum* 1992;35:835–837

34   Pernikoff BJ, Eisenstat TE, Rubin RJ, Oliver GC, Salvati EP. Reappraisal of partial lateral internal sphincterotomy. *Dis Colon Rectum* 1994;37:1291–1295

35   Garcia-Aguilar J, Belmonte C, Wong WD, Lowry AC, Madoff RD. Open *vs.* closed sphincterotomy for chronic anal fissure: long term results. *Dis Colon Rectum* 1996;39:440–443

36   Littlejohn DRG, Newstead GL. Tailored lateral sphincterotomy for anal fissure. *Dis Colon Rectum* 1997;40:1439–1442

37   Keighley MRB, Greca F, Nevah E, Hares M, Alexander-Williams J. Treatment of anal fissure by lateral subcutaneous sphincterotomy should be under general anesthesia. *Br J Surg* 1981;68:400–401

38 Sultan AH, Kamm MA, Nicholls RJ, Bartram CI. Prospective study of the extent of internal anal sphincter division during lateral anal sphincterotomy. *Dis Colon Rectum* 1994;37:1031–1033

39 Nickell WB, Woodward ER. Advancement flaps for treatment of anal stricture. *Arch Surg* 1972;104:223–224

40 Leong AFPK, Seow-Choen F. Lateral sphincterotomy compared with anal advancement flap for chronic anal fissure. *Dis Colon Rectum* 1995;38:69–71

41 Corby H, Donnelly VS, O'Herlihy C, O'Connell PR. Anal canal pressures are low in women with postpartum anal fissure. *Br J Surg* 1997;84:86–88

42 Nyam DCNK, Wilson RG, Stewart KT, Farouk R, Bartolo DCC. Island advancement flaps in the management of anal fissures. *Br J Surg* 1995;82:326–328

43 Shub HA, Salvati EP, Rubin RJ. Conservative treatment of anal fissure: an unselected retrospective and continuous study. *Dis Colon Rectum* 1978;21:582–583

44 Jensen SL. Maintenance therapy with unprocessed bran in the prevention of acute anal fissure recurrence. *J R Soc Med* 1987;80:296–298

45 Gough MJ, Lewis A. The conservative treatment of fissure-in-ano. *Br J Surg* 1983; 70:175–176

46 Motson RW, Keck JO. Pathogenesis and treatment of anal fissure. In: Henry MM, Swash M (eds) *Coloproctology and the Pelvic Floor*, 2nd edn. Butterworth-Heinemann, Oxford, UK, 1992

47 McDonald P, Driscoll AM, Nicholls RJ. The anal dilator in the conservative management of acute anal fissures. *Br J Surg* 1983;70:25–26

48 O'Kelly TJ, Brading A, Mortensen N. *In vitro* response of the human anal canal longitudinal muscle layer to cholinergic and adrenergic stimulation: evidence of sphincter specialisation. *Br J Surg* 1993;80:1337–1341

49 O'Kelly TJ, Brading A, Mortensen N. Nerve mediated relaxation of the human internal anal sphincter: the role of nitric oxide. *Gut* 1993;34:689–693

50 Schouten WR, Briel JW, Boerma MO, Auwerda JJA, Wilms EB, Graatsma BH. Pathophysiological aspects and clinical outcome of intra-anal application of isosorbide dinitrate in patients with chronic anal fissure. *Gut* 1996;39:465–469

51 Lund JN, Scholefield JF. A randomised, prospective, double-blind, placebo-controlled trial of glyceryl trinitrate ointment in treatment of anal fissure. *Lancet* 1997;349:11–14

52 Carapeti EA, Kamm MA, McDonald PJ, Chadwick, Melville D, Phillips RKS. Randomised controlled trial shows that glyceryl nitrate heals anal fissures, higher doses are not more effective, and there is a high recurrence rate. *Gut* 1999;4:727–730

53 Loder PB, Kamm MA, Nicholls RJ, Phillips RKS. 'Reversible chemical sympathectomy' by local application of glyceryl trinitrate. *Br J Surg* 1994;81:1386–1389

54 Gorfine SR. Topical nitroglycerin therapy for anal fissures and ulcers. *N Eng J Med* 1995;333:1156–1157

55 Gorfine SR. Treatment of benign anal disease with topical nitroglycerin. *Dis Colon Rectum* 1995;38:453–457

56 Lund JN, Armitage NC, Scholefield JH. Use of glyceryl trinitrate in the treatment of anal fissure. *Br J Surg* 1996;83:776–777

57  Watson SJ, Kamm MA, Nicholls RJ, Phillips RKS. Topical glyceryl trinitrate in the treatment of chronic anal fissure. *Br J Surg* 1996;**83**:771–775

58  Lund JN, Scholefield JF. Glyceryl trinitrate is an effective treatment for anal fissure. *Dis Colon Rectum* 1997;**40**:468–470

59  Bacher H, Mischinger H-J, Werkgartner G *et al*. Local nitroglycerin for treatment of anal fissures: an alternative to lateral sphincterotomy? *Dis Colon Rectum* 1997;**40**:840–845

60  Oettle GJ. Glyceryl trinitrate *vs*. sphincterotomy for treatment of chronic fissure-in-ano. A randomised controlled trial. *Dis Colon Rectum* 1997;**40**:1318–1320

61  Royal College of Surgeons of England in association with Association of Coloproctology of Great Britain and Ireland Analyses of 1997. Study on Anal Fissure in Children and Adults, London, 1998

62  Manookian CM, Fleshner P, Moore B, Cooperman H, Sokol T. Topical nitroglycerin in the management of anal fissure: an explosive outcome! *Am Surg* 1998;**64**:962–964

63  Kennedy ML, Sowter S, Nguyen H, Lubowski DZ. Glyceryl trinitrate ointment for the treatment of chronic anal fissure; results of a placebo-controlled trial and long-term follow-up. *Dis Colon Rectum* 1999;**42**:1000–1006

64  Jonas M, Lobo DN, Gudgeon AM. Lateral internal sphincterotomy is not redundant in the era of glyceryl trinitrate therapy for chronic anal fissure. *J R Soc Med* 1999;**92**:186–187

65  Hyman NH, Cataldo PA. Nitroglycerin ointment for anal fissures; effective treatment or just a headache? *Dis Colon Rectum* 1999;**42**:383–385

66  Brisinda G, Maria G, Bentivoglio AR, Cassetta E, Gui D, Albanese A. A comparison of injections of botulinum toxin and topical nitroglycerin ointment for the treatment of chronic anal fissure. *N Eng J Med* 1999;**341**:65–69

67  Pitt J, Dawas K, Dawson PM. Disappointing results of glyceryl trinitrate ointment in the treatment of chronic fissure-in-ano in a district general hospital. *Colorectal Dis* 1999;**1**:204–206

68  Dorfman G, Levitt M, Platell C. Treatment of chronic anal fissure with topical glyceryl trinitrate. *Dis Colon Rectum* 1999;**42**:1007–1010

69  Lund JN, Scholefield JH. Internal sphincter spasm in anal fissure. *Br J Surg* 1997;**84**:1723–1724

70  Lund JN, Scholefield JH. Follow-up of patients with chronic anal fissure treated with topical glyceryl trinitrate. *Lancet* 1998;**352**:1681

71  Lysy J, Israel-Yatzkan Y, Sestiere-Ittah M, Keret D, Goldin E. Treatment of chronic anal fissure with isosorbide dinitrate; long-term results and dose determination. *Dis Colon Rectum* 1998;**41**:1406–1410

72  Jankovic J, Brin MF. Therapeutic uses of botulinum toxin. *N Eng J Med* 1991;**324**:1186–1194

73  Moore AP. The management of chronic fissure in-ano with botulinum toxin. *J R Coll Surg Edin* 1997;**42**:289

74  Jost WH, Schimrigk K. Use of botulinum toxin in anal fissure (letter). *Dis Colon Rectum* 1993;**36**:974

75  Gui D, Cassetta E, Anastasio G, Bentivoglio AR, Maria G, Albanese A. Botulinum toxin for chronic anal fissure. *Lancet* 1994;**344**:1127–1128

76  Jost WH, Schimrigk K. Therapy of anal fissure using botulinum toxin. *Dis Colon Rectum* 1994;37:1321–1324

77  Jost WH, Mlitz H, Schanne S, Schimrigk K. Botulinum toxin in the treatment of fissure-in-ano. *Coloproctology* 1995;17:224–229

78  Jost WH. One hundred cases of anal fissure treated with botulinum toxin. Early and long-term results. *Dis Colon Rectum* 1997;40:1029–1032

79  Espi A, Melo F, Minguez M *et al*. Therapeutic use of botulinum toxin in anal fissure. *Int J Colorectal Dis* 1997;12:163(abstract)

80  Maria G, Cassetta E, Gui D, Brisinda G, Bentivoglio AR, Albanese A. A comparison of botulinum toxin and saline for the treatment of chronic anal fissure. *N Eng J Med* 1998;388:217–220

81  Gonzales CP, Perez RF, Legaz HML, Ruiz CK, Saez BJM. The treatment of anal fissure with botulinum toxin (Spanish) *Gastro y Hepato* 1999;22:163–166

82  Minguez M, Melo F, Espi A *et al*. Therapeutic effects of different doses of botulinum toxin in chronic anal fissure. *Dis Colon Rectum* 1999;42:1016–1021

83  Mason PF, Watkins MJG, Hall HS, Hall AW. The management of chronic fissure-in-ano with botulinum toxin. *J R Coll Surg Edin* 1996;41:235–238

84  Jost WH, Schrank B. Chronic anal fissures treated with botulinum toxin injections: a dose-finding study with Dysport®. *Colorectal Dis* 1999;1:26–28

85  Carapeti EA, Kamm MA, Phillips RKS. Topical and oral diltiazem lower the resting anal pressure. *Br J Surg* 1998;85(suppl):80

86  Carapeti EA, Kamm MA, Evans BK, Phillips RKS. Topical diltiazem and bethanecol decrease anal sphincter pressure without side-effects. *Gut* 1999;45:719–722.

87  Chrysos E, Xynos E, Tzovaras G, Zoras OJ, Tsiaoussis J, Vassilakis SJ. Effect of nifedipine on rectoanal motility. *Dis Colon Rectum* 1996;39:212–216

88  Cook TA, Humphreys MMS, Mortensen NJMcC. Oral nifedepine is an effective treatment for chronic anal fissures. *Dis Colon Rectum* 1999;42:A32(abstract)

89  Antorpoli C, Perrolti P, Rubino M *et al*. Nifedipine for local use in conservative treatment of anal fissures. *Dis Colon Rectum* 1999;42:1011–1015

90  Pitt J, Henry MM, Craggs MD, Boulos PB. A potential new medical therapy for chronic anal fissure. *Int J Colorectal Dis* 1997;12:169(abstract)

91  Ojo-Aromokudu O, Pitt J, Boulos PB, Knight SL, Craggs MD. A comparison of $\alpha$- and $\beta$-adrenoceptor function of the internal anal sphincter in people with and without chronic anal fissures. *J Physiol* 1998;507:19P

92  Catto JWF, Hinson FL, Leveson SH. Topical glyceryl trinitrate cream for anal fissure. *Br J Surg* 1998;85:874–875

# 5 Controversies in constipation: What are the treatment options?

*Johann Pfeifer and Selman Uranüs*

## INTRODUCTION

Constipation is one of the most frequent gastrointestinal symptoms and reasons for medical consultation.[1] Constipation is related to intestinal motility disorders, pelvic floor disturbance, or a combination of both; the exact origin of these disorders is unknown. The role of the surgical approach in the treatment of constipation is still controversial. This chapter is intended to define the indications and choice of treatment for chronic constipation.

## DEFINING THE CLINICAL PROBLEM

The definition of constipation includes both subjective and objective aspects, whereby physicians and patients differ in their opinions of what constitutes constipation. While most physicians consider two or fewer bowel movements per week as constipation,[2] most patients would include subjective complaints such as incomplete evacuation, abdominal or rectal pain, firm stool consistency, and need for straining. Recently, Ashraf *et al.*[3] reported that less than half of the patients who feel they are constipated are in fact so when physiologically evaluated. According to Kumar *et al.*, 'In practice…constipation presents as a problem when the patient feels the situation to be unsatisfactory. Thus, even a patient with daily bowel movements can feel constipated and require investigation'.[4]

## DEFINITION

Drossman *et al.*[5] defined constipation as two or fewer stools per week and/or straining at stool more than 25% of the time. Subsequently the best definition for constipation was proposed by Whitehead *et al.*[6] as two or more of the following complaints present when the patient is not taking laxatives, and persisting for at least 12 months: (1) straining on more than 25% of bowel movements; (2) feeling of incomplete evacuation after more than 25% of bowel movements; (3) scybalous stools on more than 25% of bowel movements; (4) stools less frequent than two per week with or without other symptoms of constipation.

A scoring system for constipation, like that for incontinence,[7] has been proposed to allow evaluation of patients and a more accurate comparison of indications and results of surgery of constipation (Table 5.1).[8]

**Table 5.1** Constipation scoring system[8]

| Measure | Score |
| --- | --- |
| Frequency of bowel movements | |
| 1–2 times per 1–2 days | 0 |
| 2 times per week | 1 |
| Once per week | 2 |
| Less than once per week | 3 |
| Less than once per month | 4 |
| Difficulty: painful evacuation effort | |
| Never | 0 |
| Rarely | 1 |
| Sometimes | 2 |
| Usually | 3 |
| Always | 4 |
| Completeness: feeling of incomplete evacuation | |
| Never | 0 |
| Rarely | 1 |
| Sometimes | 2 |
| Usually | 3 |
| Always | 4 |
| Pain: abdominal pain | |
| Never | 0 |
| Rarely | 1 |
| Sometimes | 2 |
| Usually | 3 |
| Always | 4 |

**Table 5.1** (*continued*)

| Measure | Score |
|---|---|
| Times: minutes in lavatory per attempt | |
| Less than 5 | 0 |
| 5–10 | 1 |
| 10–20 | 2 |
| 20–30 | 3 |
| More than 30 | 4 |
| Assistance: type of assistance | |
| Without assistance | 0 |
| Stimulant laxatives | 1 |
| Digital assistance or enema | 2 |
| Failure: unsuccessful attempts at evacuation per 24 hours | |
| Never | 0 |
| 1–3 | 1 |
| 3–6 | 2 |
| 6–9 | 3 |
| More than 9 | 4 |
| History: duration of constipation (years) | |
| 0 | 0 |
| 1–5 | 1 |
| 5–10 | 2 |
| 10–20 | 3 |
| More than 20 | 4 |

Minimum score: 0; maximum score: 30.

## ASSESSMENT AND INVESTIGATIONS

A detailed history addressing the specifics of bowel activity, including the need for perineal support or digitation and other gastrointestinal and systemic symptoms, is essential; a scoring system, as described above, to rate the severity of constipation is useful.[8] Some estimate of the amount and type of dietary intake and of medications that may have a constipating effect and use of laxatives, suppositories, and enemas should be elicited. Table 5.2 lists all extracolonic causes of

**Table 5.2** Extracolonic causes of constipation

Endocrine
    Diabetes mellitus
    Hyperparathyroidism
    Hypothyroidism

Metabolic
    Hypokalemia
    Hypercalcemia

Neurologic
    Cerebral
        Parkinson's disease
        Stroke
    Spinal
        Multiple sclerosis
        Trauma
    Peripheral
        Chagas' disease
        Von Recklinghausen's disease

Drugs
    Antidepressants
    Calcium channel blockers

Myopathic
    Scleroderma
    Amyloidosis

constipation that should be systematically excluded by a detailed history and examination.

## Examination

A physical examination should be conducted with attention to features of extracolonic disorders. Inspection of the anus and the perianal area can provide diagnostic clues in the form of hemorrhoids, fissures, sentinel tags, and skin changes, as well as the presence of perineal descent while bearing down. Digital examination will show if there is fecal impaction, suggestive of habitual constipation (psychogenic), or is empty due to inadequate fiber or fluid intake (functional) and in patients with Hirschsprung's disease. It also allows assessment of the sphincter tone at rest, and of the external sphincter and puborectalis tone at squeeze. The rectal size can also be appreciated. Anoscopy and proctosigmoidoscopy can demonstrate hemorrhoids, fissures, solitary rectal ulcer, intussusception, and anterior mucosal prolapse, or any associated features of constipation such as melanosis coli and will exclude neoplasms or inflammatory bowel disease. Evidence of rectocele, commonly anteriorly in females, should be sought by vaginal examination during straining.

A barium enema and/or a colonoscopy will exclude colonic dilatation and obstructive lesions such as neoplasia or strictures. In addition blood chemistry, specifically serum calcium, potassium, and thyroxine levels, will rule out endocrine or metabolic disorders. If initial comprehensive assessment fails to identify a cause, physiologic investigation is required.

## Colonic motility study

The passage of colonic contents may be delineated with indigo carmine, charcoal, barium, radioisotopes, microtelemetry units, and radiopaque markers.[9–13] The latter technique is the least expensive, easiest to perform, and most informative. The radiopaque markers are ingested, and the time to arrival in the rectum is evaluated by serial abdominal radiographs. In normal subjects 80% of the markers are passed by the fifth postingestion day and all are expelled by day 7.[12,14] If more than 20% are diffusely retained the diagnosis of colonic inertia can be made, whereas a delay in the rectosigmoid region is suggestive of pelvic floor dysfunction or of a sigmoidocele. Intraluminal measurement of colonic myoelectrical and motor function is still experimental,[15] therefore colonic transit study is the most widely used method of assessment.[16]

## Anorectal manometry

Anorectal manometry can be performed with perfused catheters, microtransducers mounted on perfused catheters, or several other devices.[17–22] This technique allows measurement of the length of the anal canal (high pressure zone) and of the resting and squeeze pressures (which is relevant should colectomy become necessary), rectal capacity, volume to first sensation and, most importantly, the rectoanal inhibitory reflex which is absent in adult short or ultrashort segment[23] and in Chagas' disease. Some patients with idiopathic megarectum may show a false-negative reflex owing to difficulty in rapidly distending the dilated rectum.

## Balloon expulsion

A latex balloon is inserted into the rectum and then filled with 50 ml of water. Patients with pelvic floor disorders require weight to expel the balloon or, sometimes, are totally unable to expel the balloon,[24] because of failure to relax the pelvic floor during attempted evacuation.

## Cinedefecography

Cinedefecography is a dynamic study to visualize the anal canal and the rectum during various phases of evacuation. A contrast medium of the consistency of stool is instilled into the rectum and radiographs are obtained with fluoroscopic control while the patient is at rest, during squeeze, while pushing, and after evacuation.[25] This test is especially useful for diagnosing dysfunctional outlet obstruction, particularly paradoxical puborectalis contraction, rectocele, rectoanal intussusception, and perineal descent. However, cinedefecography reveals abnormalities in as many as 50% of asymptomatic individuals.[26,27] Although measurement of the anorectal angle may be unreliable, when significant findings worthy of intensive conservative (biofeedback) or surgical treatment are considered alone, cinedefecographic findings are reliable and reproducible in 88% of patients.[28]

## Electromyography (EMG) and pudendal nerve terminal motor latency (PNTML)

The most common technique is placement of fine wire electrodes into the external anal sphincter and puborectalis muscle. Once in place, these wires are relatively 'painless' and do not interfere with normal evacuation. A less painful and equally reliable method using a sponge or patch electrodes has recently been described.[29] In a normal EMG continuous electrical activity at rest is increased during squeezing and coughing and returns to its resting pattern during evacuation. EMG is the best method to demonstrate paradoxical puborectalis contraction. PNTML is measured by an electrode mounted on the examiner's finger, which is placed onto the ischial spine. The time between application of the electrical stimulus and the external sphincter contraction is a measure of the terminal motor latency of the pudendal nerve.[30] However, prolonged motor latency as a prognostic marker for treatment is still controversial.[31]

## Other tests

When evaluating constipated patients, several other techniques have been proposed, including ultrasonography,[32] balloon proctography,[33] perineometry,[33] scintigraphic assessment of rectal evacuation,[34] mechanical and electrical stimulation of sensation,[35] as well as evoked potentials by rectal[36] or cerebral stimulation.[36] It is worth mentioning that no single test alone is pathognomonic, and therefore diagnosing functional disorders must be based upon several tests. In particular, when considering surgery, physiologic investigation is mandatory to optimize postoperative outcome.[37]

Esophageal manometry, gastric motility, and small-bowel transit studies have shown that there may be two different types of idiopathic slow transit constipation:[38] one type involves only the colon; and the other, the entire gastrointestinal tract. Long-term surgical results after colectomy are unfavorable in patients with total gastrointestinal dysmotility disorders compared with patients with isolated colonic slow transit constipation.[38] Patients with a panenteric dysmotility may also have changes in gastric emptying[39] and biliary function.[40] Therefore, upper gastrointestinal evaluation should be considered when colonic transit studies show colonic inertia to exclude this subgroup of patients with gastrointestinal dysmotility, particularly when an operative approach is being considered.

## INTERPRETATION OF RESULTS

The aim of diagnostic evaluation is to determine any objective abnormalities associated with constipation. Therefore, initially, extracolonic or structural disorders are excluded. If no cause for constipation is identified, a colonic transit study should be performed. If the transit study is normal, assessment of the pelvic floor should follow by cinede-fecography and EMG. After diagnostic evaluation, constipation can be categorized as follows:

1 • Colonic inertia or slow transit constipation without megabowel.
  • Colonic inertia or slow transit constipation with megabowel.
  • Colonic inertia or slow transit constipation as part of a comprehensive gut dysmotility disorder.

2 • Pelvic floor dysfunction with anatomical abnormality (Hirschsprung's disease, rectocele, sigmoidocele, intussusception, rectal prolapse).
   • Pelvic floor dysfunction without anatomical abnormality (paradoxical puborectalis contraction, levator spasm, anismus, rectal pain).
3 Combined slow transit constipation and pelvic floor dysfunction.
4 Normal transit constipation (possibly due to irritable bowel disease).

## SURGICAL TREATMENT

Surgical treatment should only be considered after intensive dietary manipulation, addition of fiber preparations, judicious laxative intake, and use of enemas and suppositories have failed. It is also essential that candidates for surgery with any history of prior psychological or psychiatric disorder should undergo preoperative psychiatric assessment.

### Colonic inertia with and without megacolon and/or megarectum

#### Colectomy
Subtotal colectomy has been the standard operation for patients with colonic inertia. Although there is no difference in treatment options, treating megabowel is surgically more challenging. Because of dilatation it is often not possible to staple the distal rectal stump; a hand-sutured anastomosis will generally be required.[41] The variance in success rates shown in Table 5.3 is related to patient selection, as unfavorable factors were not recognized during earlier experiences.

Subtotal colectomy with ileorectal, ileosigmoid, or cecorectal anastomosis has been employed. Subtotal colectomy with cecorectal anastomosis has the theoretical advantage of retaining the ileocecal valve to enhance absorption of water and to avoid severe diarrhea. However, preservation of the cecum is often complicated by cecal distension and constipation; thus, the results have been disappointing. Fasth *et al.*[51] reported success in only 25% of patients. Preston *et al.*[24] also noted a slightly higher postoperative constipation rate after cecorectal anastomosis, whereas Yoshioka & Keighley[45] found no difference between cecorectal and ileorectal anastomosis. Stabile *et al.*[52] however, recognized a functional benefit after colectomy

**Table 5.3** Subtotal colectomy with ileorectal anastomosis with or without megacolon

| Series/year | n | Female (%) | Mean age (years) | Follow up (years) | No megacolon | Success (%) | Megacolon | Success (%) |
|---|---|---|---|---|---|---|---|---|
| Preston/ 1984[24] | 8 | 100 | 26 | 5.7 | 8 | 63 | — | — |
| Barnes/ 1986[42] | 6 | 43 | 38 | 5 | — | — | 6 | 67 |
| Akervall/ 1988[43] | 12 | 100 | 39 | 3.4 | 12 | 66 | — | — |
| Kamm/ 1988[44] | 33 | 100 | 34 | 2 | 33 | 50 | — | — |
| Yoshioka/ 1989[45] | 40[a] | 98 | 35 | 3 | 32 | 58[b] | 8 | 58[b] |
| Pena/ 1992[46] | 105 | 91 | 43 | 8 | 78 | 89 | — | — |
| Takahashi/ 1994[47] | 38[c] | — | — | 3 | 37 | 97 | — | — |
| Redmond/ 1995[38] | 34 | 92 | 43 | 7.5 | 34 | 90[d] 13[e] | — | — |
| Piccirillo/ 1995[48] | 54 | 78 | 49 | 2.2 | 54 | 94 | — | — |
| Pluta/ 1996[49] | 24 | — | — | — | — | 71 | — | — |
| Nyam/ 1997[50] | 74 | 92 | 53 | 4.6 | 74 | 97 | — | — |

[a] 34 ileorectal anastomosies, 5 cecorectal anastomosies, 1 ileosigmoid anastomosis.
[b] Overall success.
[c] Ileorectal anastomosis or ileosigmoid anastomosis.
[d] For colonic inertia.
[e] For gastrointestinal dysmotility.

and ileorectal anastomosis compared with cecorectal anastomosis or sigmoid resection. Subtotal colectomy with ileosigmoid anastomosis may also fail to treat constipation. Pemberton *et al.*[53] converted 50% of patients from ileosigmoid anastomosis to ileorectal anastomosis.

Preston *et al.*[24] reported 21 female patients with radiologically normal colon and colonic inertia on colonic transit studies. At a mean follow up of 5.7 years, 10 of the 16 (63%) patients who underwent a colectomy with either ileorectal ($n = 8$) or cecorectal ($n = 8$) anastomosis were able to discontinue laxative use, noticeably among the patients who had had an ileorectal anastomosis. In the majority, rectal sensation prior to surgery was impaired. Conversely, five patients who had partial colon resections (two left hemicolectomy, three sigmoid colectomy, one with a Duhamel) remained constipated. Akervall *et al.*[43] reported 12 women with colonic inertia, seven of whom had previously undergone resection. All underwent a subtotal colectomy or completion colectomy and an ileorectal anastomosis. At a mean follow up of 3.4 years, eight (66%) patients with a preoperative normal rectal sensation had a good outcome; the four failures had impaired sensation prior to surgery. Thus, a functional improvement after subtotal colectomy and ileorectal anastomosis is more likely to be achieved in patients with normal rectal sensation. A defect in the afferent innervation of the rectum in severe constipation seems to influence the functional outcome as these patients seem to require greater pressure for sensation and sphincter relaxation.

Yoshioka & Keighley[45] reported 40 patients with colonic inertia, of whom eight patients had megacolon or megarectum and 19 patients (48%) had paradoxical puborectalis contraction: 34 patients underwent an ileorectal anastomosis, five a cecorectal anastomosis, and one an ileosigmoid anastomosis. Fourteen patients (35%) had postoperative diarrhea, four a small bowel obstruction, and one was incontinent. Twelve patients (30%) required reoperation: six had an ileostomy and six had severe postoperative constipation leading to megarectum, and were treated with protectomy and a pouch–anal anastomosis to ultimately achieve an overall satisfaction rate of 58%. In 1988 Kamm *et al.*[44] retrospectively assessed 44 women; in 35 of 36 patients, a colonic transit study revealed prolonged transit; 13 of the 20 patients who underwent EMG showed paradoxical puborectalis contraction pattern; and 21 of 29 patients failed the balloon expulsion test. Subtotal colectomy was performed with ileorectal anastomosis in 33 patients and a cecorectal anastomosis in 11 patients. At 3-years follow up, successful outcome was reported by 22 patients (50%); 17 (39%) had diarrhea, five (11%) recurrent constipation, and 20 (45%) continued to use laxatives. Ten patients (23%) had a reoperation – an ileostomy in six, puborectalis division in three, and puborectalis division with a Delorme resection in one patient.

Hence, the failure of subtotal colectomy in these reports must be attributable to concomitant pelvic floor dysfunction as the anticipated success rate of surgical treatment for isolated colonic inertia is higher. Indeed, Vasilevsky *et al.*[54] presented 51 consecutive severely constipated patients evaluated by colonic transit study in 30 and anorectal manometry in 16; all underwent barium enema or colonoscopy which demonstrated a megacolon in 14 patients. Forty-six patients had a subtotal colectomy with an ileosigmoid anastomosis and five had an ileorectal anastomosis. The overall satisfaction rate at a median follow up of 4 years was 81%; in another study by the same group the satisfaction rate was 89% at 8 years in 105 patients.[46] Similarly, Piccirillo *et al.*[48] achieved 94% successful outcomes after subtotal colectomy with ileorectal anastomosis in 54 patients who had colonic inertia defined by a colonic transit study and without paradoxical puborectalis contraction on cinedefecography or EMG at a mean follow up of 27 months. Conversely, in the Mayo Clinic series[50] of 68 females and six males with a mean age of 53, the success rate for subtotal colectomy and ileorectal anastomosis was 97% at a mean follow up of 56 months. However, the authors failed to identify any differences in outcome for patients with ($n = 22$) or without ($n = 52$) concomitant pelvic floor dysfunction.

Pluta *et al.*[49] reported good or excellent results in 17 (71%) of 24 patients after subtotal colectomy and ileorectal anastomosis. In this series psychiatric illness did correlate with the outcome. An excellent or much improved result was seen in 13 of 14 patients with no psychiatric history but only in four of 10 patients with a psychiatric history. Severity of illness was a significant predictor. Furthermore, as observed by others,[24,43] patients with diminished rectal sensitivity had a poorer result.

In an interesting contribution by Redmond *et al.*,[38] 37 patients with constipation underwent physiologic and radiologic evaluation of the upper and lower gastrointestinal tract. In this series 21 patients (18 females, three males) were found to have isolated colonic inertia (CI) and the remaining 16 female patients had gastrointestinal dysmotility (GID) with colonic predominance. Thirty-four patients underwent a subtotal colectomy with ileorectal anastomosis and three a subtotal colectomy with an end ileostomy. At a mean follow up of 7.5 years, three died due to unrelated causes. In the CI group, the bowel frequency increased from 1.7 per week preoperatively to 36 per week after 6 months, then diminished to 23 per week after 1 year and remained constant for up to 10 years. Thus, CI patients had a successful long-term outcome of 90%. In comparison, after 1 year 12%, and within 5 years 80% of the patients with GID were constipated.

## Segmental colonic resection

Segmental resection of the colon has been associated with poor outcome and results in recurrent constipation possibly due, in part, to dilatation of the remaining colon. However, its role for colonic inertia when not associated with a megabowel is debatable.

Gray & Marteinsson[55] had no success in all four patients with colonic inertia and Preston et al.[24] reported the same failure rate in five patients: in two of these, partial left-sided colectomy was performed, and in three, sigmoid resection. However, Kamm et al.[44] reported successful outcome in two female patients who were investigated by colonic transit study, balloon expulsion test, anorectal manometry, and cinedefecography. A left colectomy with a distal rectal anastomosis was performed on one patient and a coloanal anastomosis on the other: patients were well at 2 and 3 years after surgery, respectively. With this limited experience, Kamm et al. concluded that in a carefully selected subgroup of patients this operation may provide better symptomatic results than colectomy with ileorectal anastomosis.

DeGraaf et al.,[56] on the basis of segmental colonic transit times, selected 24 patients for subtotal colectomy and 18 for left-sided segmental resection. Subtotal colectomy was advised when the progression of markers was delayed in all segments of the colon and partial left-sided colectomy when transit in the right colon was normal. After left-sided colectomy and subtotal colectomy, 12 (66%) of 18 patients and 15 (62%) of 24, respectively, expressed satisfaction with the outcome. Recurrent constipation was seen in three (16%) of 18 and seven (30%) of 24; severe abdominal discomfort was noted in six (33%) of 18 and 15 (75%) of 24; disabling diarrhea and fecal incontinence developed in two (14%) of 14 and five (25%) of 20 patients, respectively. The authors believed that evaluation of clinical outcome should be based on all the above criteria, as these may diminish the quality of life. In this respect there is, therefore, an advantage in segmental resection but the authors point out that both procedures should be selected with prudence.

## Surgery for megabowel

The reported results of surgery for megabowel are confusing. Most studies are retrospective, and there is uncertainty about the underlying abnormality because physiologic investigations are lacking. Stabile et al.[57] reported on seven patients (two females, five males) of a mean age of 19 years; one patient had previously had a Duhamel operation. All patients had a megarectum and megasigmoid and underwent partial colectomy with coloanal anastomosis. One patient died and two developed a postoperative pelvic abscess and a rectovaginal fistula; only four patients showed good results. This compares unfavorably with the results obtained in another report from the same group.[42] In a series of 40 patients – with idiopathic megarectum and megabowel following colectomy and cecorectal anastomosis in 22 patients, colectomy and ileorectal anastomosis in 11, and sigmoid resection in seven – 35 (83%) had normal bowel function, none had recurrent constipation after ileorectal anastomosis, one patient died, and four required subsequent laparotomy for bowel obstruction.

The role of rectal excision using the Soave, Duhamel, or the Swenson pull-through techniques is still controversial as such reports are only sporadic (Table 5.4). Parc *et al.*[58] reported a series of patients with megabowel treated by the Duhamel technique, with a good functional outcome in 32 of 34 patients, with no mortality and a reasonable morbidity, consisting of two pelvic abscesses, five anastomotic strictures, and one conservatively treated bowel obstruction. Stabile *et al.*[59] reported suboptimal results in 20 patients with megabowel, only half achieving normal bowel frequency after a Duhamel operation. Three patients had a pelvic abscess, five patients had a fecal fistula, and one patient had a rectovaginal fistula. Furthermore, five of seven patients who remained constipated required further surgery.

**Table 5.4** Abdominal procedures for Hirschsprung's disease[70]

| Surgical method | Success (%) | Minor complications (%) | Major complications (%) | Remarks |
|---|---|---|---|---|
| Duhamel | 91 | 2 | 10 | Avoids pelvic dissection |
| Swenson | 80 | 7 | 33 | 7% incidence of impotence |
| Soave | 85 | 13 | 25 | 13% postoperative stricture 16% anastomotic leak rate |

Sigmoid resection is probably the optimal procedure for idiopathic megasigmoid: Hughes *et al.*[60] noted satisfactory results in all five patients in their series; Belliveau *et al.*[61] in six of seven patients (86%); McCready *et al.*[62] in six of eight patients (75%); and Coremans[63] in both patients with a megasigmoid. The procedure is especially promising when there is a long sigmoid colon with a predisposition for volvulus formation. Lane & Todd,[64] however, reported success in only one of six patients (17%) with a megasigmoid but who also had a megarectum.

It seems that for patients with a moderately dilated rectum or dilated colon, colectomy and ileorectal anastomosis offers the best result. In those patients with a grossly dilated rectum and distal colon, the Duhamel operation must be considered, because it involves excision of most of the dilated segment. However, the results are not as uniformly satisfactory in this group of patients as those in patients with adult Hirschsprung's disease.

Therefore, the distinction between idiopathic megabowel and adult Hirschsprung's disease is crucial, since between 25 and 50% of megabowel will not be due to Hirschsprung's disease. The diagnosis is confirmed by the absence of ganglia in a full-thickness biopsy or anorectal myectomy which may possibly treat short or ultrashort segment Hirschsprung's disease. Posterior anorectal myectomy is performed by removing a 1 cm wide and at least 6 cm long strip of internal anal sphincter and circular muscle, starting 2 cm above the dentate line. Hamdy & Scobie[65] reported good results in six patients of a mean age of 21 years. In two patients on whom anorectal myectomy failed, there was improvement after a low anterior resection. Fishbein *et al.*[66] also successfully treated two patients, although the myectomy had to be doubled in length.

Standard surgical procedures for definitive treatment of Hirschsprung's disease include the Swenson abdominoperineal pull-through technique, the Duhamel retrorectal transanal anastomosis (with Martin's modification), and the Soave endorectal pull-through technique. Excision of a defined pathologic segment validates this approach and explains the satisfactory results achieved.

Elliott & Todd[67] reported the results of 39 patients (26 male, 13 female) with a mean age of 23.1 years who underwent the Duhamel procedure; 13 patients had undergone previous surgeries, five had undergone a colostomy, and three had a failed Swenson operation. The diagnosis was confirmed in all patients by full-thickness biopsy. The rectoanal inhibitory reflex was absent in 26 patients and, interestingly, present in two. Of 26 patients, a barium enema demonstrated a narrow segment in 11. Excellent functional results were achieved in 92%. Postoperative anastomotic complications were seen in 13 patients; there was no mortality. A similar experience was reported by Natsikas and Sbarounis:[68] all six patients (five males, one female) had normal bowel function, continence, and sexual function postoperatively. Luukkonen *et al.*[69] used the Duhamel procedure in seven patients and the Soave procedure in one; although postoperatively their bowel frequency was normal, five patients had episodes of incontinence. Wheatley *et al.*[70] performed four Soave procedures with good long-term success; however, one patient who underwent a Duhamel operation had to undergo further surgery because of constipation secondary to retained colorectal septum.

### Restorative proctocolectomy

Although radical, this surgical approach has been employed in patients with intractable constipation. Nicholls & Kamm[71] applied this technique to two women who refused an ileostomy; both patients had persistent constipation after subtotal colectomy. Postoperatively, one patient had spontaneous bowel movements two to three times per day and the other was improved but still required self-catheterization for complete pouch evacuation; both patients continued to have intermittent abdominal discomfort.

Stewart *et al.*[72] recently reported 34 patients with idiopathic megarectum and megacolon; 18 had megarectum and megasigmoid, one had megacolon, and 15 had megarectum and megacolon. Eight patients underwent a straight low colorectal anastomosis, two a coloanal anastomosis, eight a colonic pouch anal anastomosis, and 14 a restorative proctocolectomy with creation of an ileoanal J pouch; one patient underwent a subtotal colectomy with ileorectal anastomosis and one a loop ileostomy. One patient died 2 years after the procedure due to inhalation pneumonia complicating a small-bowel obstruction. In those patients with a straight colorectal or coloanal anastomosis, eight (44%) were continent and constipation recurred in two. One was treated with an ileostomy and the other subsequently underwent ileoanal J pouch with a stool frequency of 2–6 per day. In the colonic J-pouch group, one pouch was excised and one patient had an ileostomy because of recurrent soiling. Twelve (86%) of the 14 patients who underwent ileoanal J pouch were continent, one had recurrent soiling, and one was incontinent and subsequently required a stimulated graciloplasty. Four patients became dissatisfied because of persistent pain and ultimately underwent pouch excision. Wexner *et al.*[37] reported one young patient with colonic inertia who had undergone a low anterior resection for a Dukes' B rectal cancer 5 years earlier. This patient was free of malignancy and underwent a successful ileoanal J-pouch anastomosis.

Although a J pouch is seldom indicated, it may be useful in a few carefully selected patients, particularly those with megarectum or megacolon.

## Complications

Complications such as bleeding, anastomotic leakage, and wound infection may occur after any bowel procedure. However, the most frequent complication in patients who have undergone colectomy for constipation is small-bowel obstruction. In a review of 25 publications, Pfeifer *et al.*[73] reported an 18% overall small-bowel obstruction, 12% of whom required surgical therapy. Recent advances in adhesion prevention have included the development of a composite bioresorbable membrane of sodium hyalurinate and carboxymethylcellulose (Seprafilm®, Genzyme Corp., Cambridge, MA). In a prospective randomized surgeon-blinded series of 183 patients undergoing ileal pouch anal anastomosis, a 50% reduction in the incidence of adhesions was noted compared with the control group.[74] Similar decreases in the severity and extent of adhesions were also noted.

## Pelvic floor dysfunction with anatomic abnormality

### Rectocele

A significant rectocele is generally defined as one larger than 2 cm, as seen on cinedefecography, that does not empty by the end of the examination.[75] When a rectocele is the sole cause for outlet obstruction, as confirmed by physiologic tests, the success rate of surgical repair is reportedly very good[76] (Table 5.5). According to some authors, transvaginal repair does not provide sufficient relief[77–79] and, therefore, a combined rectovaginal or endorectal approach has been recommended. However, Sehapayak[79] reported a lower infection rate with transrectal compared with a combined procedure. Sullivan *et al.*[77] were the first to describe a transrectal rectocele repair and reported a success rate of 97.5% in 151 patients. Sehapayak[79] reported

**Table 5.5** Surgery for rectocele

| Series/year | n | Success (%) | Surgical approach |
| --- | --- | --- | --- |
| Sullivan/1968[77] | 151 | 97.5 | Transrectal |
| Capps/1975[78] | 50 | 76 | Transrectal |
| Sehapayak/1985[79] | 355 | 98 | Transrectal |
| Janssen/1994[80] | 76 | 92 | Transrectal |
| Mellgren/1995[82] | 25 | 88 | Transvaginal |
| Murthy/1996[81] | 33 | 92 | Transrectal (31) Transabdominal (2) |

an improvement of 98% in 355 women with a mean age of 50 years after a transrectal repair. Janssen and Van Dijke[80] had a good result in 92% of 76 women and Murthy *et al.*[81] had a similar experience in 33 patients. In 25 patients reported by Mellgren *et al.*,[82] a transvaginal repair by posterior perineorrhaphy and colporrhaphy produced improved symptoms in 21 patients (84%); three of 16 sexually active females complained of dyspareunia.

## Sigmoidocele

Isolated sigmoidoceles which cause pelvic outlet obstruction can be classified according to the proximity of the sigmoidocele to the pelvic floor as seen on cinedefecography: first (above the pubococcygeal line), second (between the pubococcygeal and the ischiococcygeal line), and third (below the ischiococcygeal line). Five of eight patients with a third-degree and one of seven with a second-degree sigmoidocele underwent colonic resection: five had sigmoidectomy and one had subtotal colectomy because of concomitant colonic inertia. While the remaining patients with second- or third-degree sigmoidocele were managed conservatively with an improvement in only two patients, all six patients who underwent surgery reported excellent results at a mean follow up of 23 months.[83]

## Anorectal intussusception

Intussusception is often very difficult to diagnose and can be seen only on cinedefecography. It is thought that the infolding of the rectal wall obstructs the anal canal. Patients commonly feel incomplete evacuation and the sensation of a fecal bolus results in excessive straining, which further aggravates the symptoms.

Abdominal rectopexy rarely improves long-term symptomatic resolution, although some reports are encouraging. Hoffman *et al.*[84] applied a modified Ripstein procedure in eight females, with total success. Kuijpers & de Morree[85] also reported success in all 10 patients with the Wells' technique. Ihre & Seligson[86] achieved only a 64% success rate, at a mean follow up of 5 years in 39 patients, and Roe *et al.*[35] achieved a success rate of 43%. Berman *et al.*[87] investigated 21 female patients with endoscopy and cinedefecography prior to Delorme's transrectal excision: the mean follow up was 3 years, with a success rate of 70%. In the failed group, they found that intussusception was often associated with other pelvic floor disorders, such as slow transit constipation, enterocele, redundant colon, levator syndrome, anismus, and irritable bowel syndrome. Only intensive physiologic testing will provide good final results.

### Perineal descent

The exact etiology of perineal descent is unknown. At the present time there is no surgical option, although biofeedback[88] or artificial devices[89] to support the pelvic floor during defecation may improve the symptoms.

## Pelvic floor dysfunction without anatomic abnormality

### Paradoxical puborectalis contraction

In 1964 Wasserman[90] reported 75% success in four patients after a posterior partial V-shaped resection of the puborectalis muscle for puborectalis syndrome. Wallace & Madden[91] reported a similar success rate in 44 patients. However, Keighley[92] reported success in only one of seven patients after partial division of the puborectalis muscle. Similarly, Barnes *et al.*[93] reported success in only two (24%) of nine patients. Kamm *et al.*[44] and Kawano *et al.*[94] reported success rates of 24% and 43% in 18 and seven patients, respectively. Although Yu[95] had a success rate of 83% in 18 patients, most reports favor a conservative approach to paradoxical puborectalis contraction such as biofeedback therapy[96] and botulinum toxin A injection.[97]

### Levator spasm, anismus, rectal pain

Currently, there are no acceptable surgical treatment options for these entities. Although anorectal myectomy has been applied in patients with outlet obstruction, it is not a treatment that should be entertained. Pinho *et al.*[98] recently reviewed 63 patients who had undergone the procedure and who had been followed up for a mean of 30 months. Spontaneous rectal evacuation was achieved in only 17%, and 10% suffered mild incontinence. This is no longer a recommended therapy.

### Combined slow transit constipation and pelvic floor dysfunction

Several published reports already discussed[44,45] clearly demonstrate the failure of subtotal colectomy and ileorectal anastomosis when there is concomitant pelvic floor dysfunction. Biofeedback is the treatment of choice, although recent reports have documented success with botulinum toxin A injection.[99] After successful treatment of pelvic floor dysfunction by either modality, surgical treatment of an associated colonic inertia, rectocele, or sigmoidocele may further enhance the outcome.

### Normal transit constipation (probably due to irritable bowel disease)

At the moment no surgical option is routinely advised.

## CONCLUSION

Patients with intractable chronic constipation should be evaluated with physiologic testing after exclusion of extracolonic causes and psychologic assessment. Subtotal colectomy with ileorectal anastomosis is the treatment of choice for colonic inertia. Segmental colonic resection is the appropriate option for isolated megasigmoid, sigmoidocele, or recurrent sigmoid volvulus. Generally, patients with gastrointestinal dysmotility are not candidates for surgery and patients with psychiatric disorders should not be generally considered for colonic resection. Patients must be counseled that pain and/or bloating will probably persist, even if surgery normalizes bowel frequency and eliminates the need for laxatives and enemas. In most cases pelvic floor dysfunction can be treated successfully with a conservative approach.

A potential outcome of surgery for constipation is the ultimate need for a stoma. A stoma may be preferentially offered as an initial measure to patients with psychiatric disorders, inertia combined with refractory pelvic outlet obstruction, and significant pain and/or bloating. Patients who remain constipated after colectomy may well prefer a functioning stoma to a non-functioning anus.

# REFERENCES

1   Sonnenberg A, Koch TR. Epidemiology of constipation in the United States. *Dis Colon Rectum* 1989;**32**:1–8

2   Shouten WR, De Graaf JR. Severe, long standing constipation in adults: indications for surgical treatment. *Neth J Surg* 1991;**43**:222–229

3   Ashraf W, Park F, Lof J, Quigley EM. An examination of the reliability of reported stool frequency in the diagnosis of idiopathic constipation. *Am J Gastroenterol* 1996;**91**:26–32

4   Kumar D, Bartolo DCC, Devroede G *et al*. Symposium on constipation. *Int J Colorectal Dis* 1992;**7**:47–67

5   Drossman DA, Sandler RS, McKee DC, Lovitz AJ. Bowel patterns among subjects not seeking health care. *Gastroenterology* 1982;**83**:529–534

6   Whitehead WE, Chaussade S, Corazziari E, Kumar D. Report of an international workshop on management of constipation. *Int Gastroenterol* 1991;**4**:99–114

7   Jorge JM, Wexner SD. Etiology and management of fecal incontinence. *Dis Colon Rectum* 1993;**36**:77–97

8   Agachan F, Chen T, Pfeifer J, Reissman P, Wexner SD. A constipation scoring system to simplify evaluation and management of constipated patients. *Dis Colon Rectum* 1996;**39**:681–685

9   Martelli H, Devroede G, Ahran P *et al*. Some parameters of large bowel motility in normal man. *Gastroenterology* 1978;**75**:612–618

10  Kirwin WO, Smith AN. Colonic propulsion in diverticular disease, idiopathic constipation, and the irritable colon syndrome. *Scand J Gastroenterol* 1977;**12**: 331–335

11  Waller SL. Differential measurement of small and large bowel transit times in constipation and diarrhea: a new approach. *Gut* 1975;**17**:372–378

12  Hinton JM, Lennard-Jones JE, Young AC. A new method for studying gut transit times using a radiopaque marker. *Gut* 1969;**10**:842–847

13  Metcalf AM, Phillips SF, Zinsmeister AR, McCarty RL, Beart RW, Wolff BG. Simplified assessment of segmental colonic transit. *Gastroenterology* 1987;**92**:40–47

14  Ahran P, Devroede G, Jehannin B *et al*. Segmental colonic transit time. *Dis Colon Rectum* 1981;**24**:625–629

15  Camillieri M, Thompson WG, Fleshman JW, Pemberton JH. Clinical management of intractable constipation. *Ann Intern Med* 1994;**121**:520–528

16   Karulf RE, Coller JA, Bartolo DC *et al*. Anorectal physiology testing: a survey of availability and use. *Dis Colon Rectum* 1991;**34**:464–468

17   Jorge JM, Wexner SD. A practical guide to basic anorectal physiology investigations. *Contemp Surg* 1993;**43**:214–224

18   Dent OF, Goulston KJ, Zubrzycki J, Chapius PH. Bowel symptoms in an apparently well population. *Dis Colon Rectum* 1986;**29**:243–247

19   Bubrick MP, Godec CJ, Cass AS. Functional evaluation of the rectal ampullo-metrogram. *J R Soc Med* 1980;**73**:234–237

20   Molnar D, Taitz LS, Urwin OM, Wales JK. Anorectal manometry results in defecation disorders. *Arch Dis Child* 1983;**58**:257–261

21   Scharli AF, Kiesewetter WB. Defecation and continence: some new concepts. *Dis Colon Rectum* 1970;**13**:81–107

22   Rosenberg AJ, Vela AR. A new simplified technique for pediatric anorectal manometry. *Pediatrics* 1983;**71**:240–245

23   Taylor BM, Beart RW Jr, Phillips SF. Longitudinal and radial variations of pressure in the human anal sphincter. *Gastroenterology* 1984;**86**:693–697

24   Preston DM, Hawley PR, Lennard-Jones JE, Todd IP. Results of colectomy for severe idiopathic constipation in women. *Br J Surg* 1984;**71**:547–552

25   Mahieu P, Pringot J, Bodart P. Defecography I: description of a new procedure and results in normal patients. *Gastrointest Radiol* 1984;**9**:247–251

26   Goei R. Anorectal function in patients with defecation disorders and asymptomatic subjects: evaluation with defecography. *Radiology* 1990;**174**:121–123

27   Goei R, van Engelshoven J, Schouten H, Baeten C, Stassen C. Anorectal function: defecographic measurement in asymptomatic subjects. *Radiology* 1989;**173**:137–141

28   Pfeifer J, Oliveira L, Park UC, Gonzalez A, Agachan F, Wexner SD. Are interpretations of video defecographies reliable and reproducible? *Int J Colorectal Dis* 1997;**12**:67–72

29   Pfeifer J, Teoh T-A, Salanga VD, Agachan F, Wexner SD. Comparative study between intra-anal sponge and needle electrode for electromyographic evaluation of constipated patients. *Dis Colon Rectum* 1998;**41**:1153–1157

30   Henry MM, Snooks SJ, Barnes PR, Swash M. Investigation of disorders of the anorectum and colon. *Ann R Coll Surg Engl* 1985;**67**:355–360

31   Pfeifer J, Salanga VD, Agachan F, Weiss EG, Wexner SD. Variation in pudendal nerve terminal motor latency according to disease. *Dis Colon Rectum* 1997;**40**:79–83

32   Bartram CI. Anal endosonography. *Ann Gastroenterol Hepatol (Paris)* 1992;**28**:185–189

33   Henry MM, Parks AG, Swash M. The pelvic floor musculature in the descending perineum syndrome. *Br J Surg* 1982;**69**:470–472

34   O'Connell PR, Kelly KA, Brown M. Scintigraphic assessment of neorectal motor function. *J Nucl Med* 1986;**27**:460–464

35   Roe AM, Bartolo DC, Mortensen NJ. New method for assessment of anal sensation in various anorectal disorders. *Br J Surg* 1986;**73**:310–312

36    Herdmann J, Bielefeldt K, Enck P. Quantification of motor pathways to the pelvic floor in humans. *Am J Physiol* 1991;**260**:20–23

37    Wexner SD, Daniel N, Jagelman DG. Colectomy for constipation: physiologic investigation is the key to success. *Dis Colon Rectum* 1991;34:851–856

38    Redmond JM, Smith GW, Barofsky I, Ratych RE, Goldsborough DC, Schuster M. Physiological tests to predict long term outcome of total abdominal colectomy for intractable constipation. *Am J Gastroenterol* 1995;**90**:748–753

39    MacDonald A, Sunderland GT. Ambulatory manometric examination in patients with a colonic J pouch and in normal controls (letter; comment). *Br J Surg* 1997;**84**: 1031–1032

40    Hemingway D, Flett M, McKee RF, Finlay IG. Sphincter function after transanal endoscopic microsurgical excision of rectal tumors. *Dis Colon Rectum* 1996;**83**: 51–52

41    Hosie KB, Kmiot WA, Keighley MR. Constipation: another indication for restorative proctocolectomy. *Br J Surg* 1990;**77**:801–802

42    Barnes PR, Lennard-Jones JE, Hawley PR, Todd IP. Hirschsprung's disease and idiopathic megacolon in adults and adolescents. *Gut* 1986;**27**:534–541

43    Akervall S, Fasth S, Nordgren S, Oreslund T, Hulten L. The functional results after colectomy and ileorectal anastomosis for severe constipation (Arbuthnot Lane's disease) as related to rectal sensory function. *Int J Colorectal Dis* 1988;**3**: 96–101

44    Kamm MA, Hawley PR, Lennard-Jones JE. Outcome of colectomy for severe idiopathic constipation. *Gut* 1988;**29**:969–973

45    Yoshioka K, Keighley MR. Clinical results of colectomy for severe constipation. *Br J Surg* 1989;**76**:600–604

46    Pena JP, Heine JA, Wong WD, Christenson CE, Balcos EG. Subtotal colectomy for constipation – a long term follow up study [meeting abstract]. *Dis Colon Rectum* 1992;**35**:P19

47    Takahashi T, Fitzgerald SD, Pemberton JH. Evaluation and treatment of constipation. *Rev Gastroenterol Mex* 1994;**59**:133–138

48    Piccirillo MF, Reissman P, Carnavos R, Wexner SD. Colectomy as treatment for constipation in selected patients. *Br J Surg* 1995;**82**:898–901

49    Pluta H, Bowes KL, Jewell LD. Long-term results of total abdominal colectomy for chronic idiopathic constipation. Value of preoperative assessment. *Dis Colon Rectum* 1996;**39**:160–166

50    Nyam DC, Pemberton JH, Ilstrup DM, Rath DM. Long-term results of surgery for chronic constipation. *Dis Colon Rectum* 1997;**40**:273–279

51    Fasth S, Hedlund H, Svaninger G, Oreslund T, Hulten L. Functional results after subtotal colectomy and caecorectal anastomosis. *Acta Chir Scand* 1983;**149**: 623–627

52    Stabile G, Kamm MA, Hawley PR, Lennard-Jones JE. Colectomy for idiopathic megarectum and megacolon. *Gut* 1991;**32**:1538–1540

53    Pemberton JH, Rath DM, Ilstrup DM. Evaluation and surgical treatment of severe chronic constipation. *Ann Surg* 1991;**214**:403–413

54 Vasilevsky CA, Nemer FD, Balcos EG, Christenson CE, Goldberg SM. Is subtotal colectomy a viable option in the management of chronic constipation? *Dis Colon Rectum* 1988;**31**:679–681

55 Gray EJ, Marteinsson TH. Dolichocolon: indications for operations. *Am Surg* 1971; 37:509–511 (left-sided colectomy)

56 DeGraaf EJR, Gilberts LAM, Schouten WR. Role of colonic transit time studies to select patients with slow transit constipation for partial left-sided or subtotal colectomy. *Br J Surg* 1996;**83**:648–651

57 Stabile G, Kamm MA, Phillips RK, Hawley RP, Lennard-Jones JE. Partial colectomy and coloanal anastomosis for idiopathic megarectum and megacolon. *Dis Colon Rectum* 1992;**35**:158–162

58 Parc R, Berrod JL, Tussiot J, Loygue J. Le megacolon de l'adulte: a propos de 76 cas. *Ann Gastroenterol Hepatol (Paris)* 1984;**20**:133–141

59 Stabile G, Kamm MA, Hawley PR, Lennard-Jones JE. Results of the Duhamel operation on the treatment of idiopathic megarectum and megacolon. *Br J Surg* 1991;**78**:661–663

60 Hughes ES, McDermott FT, Johnson WR, Polglase AC. Surgery for constipation. *Aust NZ J Surg* 1981;**51**:144–148

61 Belliveau P, Goldberg SM, Rothenberger DA, Nivatvongs S. Idiopathic acquired megacolon: the value of subtotal colectomy. *Dis Colon Rectum* 1982;**25**:118–121

62 McCready RA, Grace RH, Todd IP. Organic constipation in adults. *Br J Surg* 1977; **64**:305–310

63 Coremans GE. Surgical aspects of severe chronic non-Hirschsprung's constipation. *Hepatogastroenterology* 1990;**37**:588–595

64 Lane RH, Todd IP. Idiopathic megacolon: a review of 42 cases. *Br J Surg* 1977;**64**: 305–310

65 Hamdy MH, Scobie WG. Anorectal myectomy in adult Hirschsprung's disease: a report of six cases. *Br J Surg* 1984;**71**:611–613

66 Fishbein RH, Handelsman JC, Schuster MM. Surgical treatment of Hirschsprung's disease in adults. *Surg Gynecol Obstet* 1986;**163**:458–464

67 Elliot MS, Todd IP. Adult Hirschsprung's disease: results of Duhamel procedure. *Br J Surg* 1985;**72**:884–885

68 Natsikas NB, Sbarounis CN. Adult Hirschsprung's disease: an experience with the Duhamel–Martin procedure with special reference to obstructed patients. *Dis Colon Rectum* 1987;**30**:204–206

69 Luukkonen P, Heikkinen M, Huikuri K, Jarvinen H. Adult Hirschsprung's disease: clinical features and functional outcome after surgery. *Dis Colon Rectum* 1990;**33**: 65–69

70 Wheatley MJ, Welsey JR, Coran AG, Polley TZ Jr. Hirschsprung's disease in adolescents and adults. *Dis Colon Rectum* 1990;**33**:662–669

71 Nicholls RJ, Kamm MA. Proctocolectomy with restorative ileoanal reservoir for severe idiopathic constipation: report of two cases. *Dis Colon Rectum* 1988;**31**: 968–969

72 Stewart J, Kumar D, Keighley MR. Results of anal low rectal anastomosis and pouch construction for megarectum and megacolon. *Br J Surg* 1994;**81**:1051–1053

73   Pfeifer J, Agachan F, Wexner SD. Surgery for constipation. A review. *Dis Colon Rectum* 1996;**39**:444–460

74   Becker JM, Dayton MT, Fazio VW *et al*. Sodium hyaluronate-based bioresorbable membrane in the prevention of postoperative abdominal adhesions: a prospective randomized double-blinded multicentered study. *J Am Coll Surg* 1996;**183**:297–306

75   Bartram CI, Turnbull GK, Lennard-Jones JE. Evacuation proctography: an investigation of rectal expulsion in 20 subjects without defecatory disturbance. *Gastrointest Radiol* 1988;**12**:72–80

76   Delemarre JB, Kruyt RH, Doornbos J *et al*. Anterior rectocele: assessment of radiographic defecography: dynamic MRI examination. *Dis Colon Rectum* 1994;**37**:249–253

77   Sullivan ES, Leaverton GH, Hardwick CE. Transrectal perineal repair: an adjunct to improved function after anorectal surgery. *Dis Colon Rectum* 1968;**11**:106–114

78   Capps WF Jr. Rectoplasty and perineoplasty for the symptomatic rectocele: a report of fifty cases. *Dis Colon Rectum* 1975;**18**:237–243

79   Sehapayak S. Transrectal repair of rectocele: an extended armamentarium of colorectal surgeons: a report of 355 cases. *Dis Colon Rectum* 1985;**28**:422–433

80   Janssen LW, van Dijke CF. Selection criteria for anterior rectal wall repair in symptomatic rectocele and anterior rectal wall prolapse. *Dis Colon Rectum* 1994;**37**:1100–1107

81   Murthy VK, Orkin BA, Smith LE, Glessman LM. Excellent outcome using selective criteria for rectocele repair. *Dis Colon Rectum* 1996;**39**:374–378

82   Mellgren A, Anzen B, Nilsson B-Y *et al*. Results of rectocele repair: a prospective study. *Dis Colon Rectum* 1995;**38**:7–13

83   Jorge JM, Yang Y-K, Wexner SD. Incidence and clinical significance of sigmoidoceles as determined by a new classification system. *Dis Colon Rectum* 1994;**37**:1112–1117

84   Hoffman MJ, Kodner IJ, Fry RD. Internal intussusception of the rectum. Diagnosis and surgical management. *Dis Colon Rectum* 1984;**27**:435–441

85   Kuijpers JH, de Morree H. Intussusception of the rectum: imagination or reality? *Ned Tijschr Geneesk* 1986;**130**:590–592

86   Ihre T, Seligson U. Intussusception of the rectum-internal procidentia: treatment and results in 90 patients. *Dis Colon Rectum* 1975;**18**:391–396

87   Berman IR, Harns MS, Rabeter MB. Delorme's transrectal excision for internal rectal prolapse. Patient selection, technique and 3 year follow up. *Dis Colon Rectum* 1990;**33**:573–580

88   Park UC, Choi SK, Piccirillo MF, Verzaro R, Wexner SD. Patterns of anismus and the relation to biofeedback therapy. *Dis Colon Rectum* 1996;**39**:768–773

89   Lesaffer LPA. Defecography update 1994. *Gent Story-Scientia* 1994;75–80

90   Wasserman IF. Puborectalis syndrome rectal stenosis due to anorectal spasm. *Dis Colon Rectum* 1964;**7**:87–98

91   Wallace WC, Madden WM. Experience with partial resection of the puborectalis muscle. *Dis Colon Rectum* 1969;**12**:196–200

92   Keighley MR. Surgery for constipation. *Br J Surg* 1998;**75**:625–626

93 Barnes PR, Hawley PR, Presto DM, Lennard-Jones JE. Experience of posterior division of the puborectalis muscle in the management of chronic constipation. *Br J Surg* 1985;**72**:475–477

94 Kawano M, Fujiyoshi T, Takagi K *et al.* Puborectalis syndrome. *J Jap Soc Coloproctol* 1987;**40**:612

95 Yu D-H. Surgical treatment of puborectalis hypertrophy. In: Wexner SD, Bartolo DC (eds) *Constipation: Etiology, Evaluation and Management.* Butterworth-Heinemann, Oxford, 1995, pp 232–239

96 Gilliland R, Heymen S, Altomare DF, Park UC, Vickers D, Wexner SD. Outcome and predictors of success of biofeedback for constipation. *Br J Surg* 1997;**84**:1123–1126

97 Jost WH. 100 cases of anal fissure treated with botulinum toxin: early and long term results. *Dis Colon Rectum* 1997;**40**:1029–1032

98 Pinho M, Yoshioka K, Keighley MR. Long-term results of anorectal myectomy for chronic constipation. *Br J Surg* 1991;**76**:1163–1164

99 Joo JS, Agachan F, Wolff B, Nogueras JJ, Wexner SD. Initial North American experience with botulinum type A for treatment of anismus. *Dis Colon Rectum* 1996;**39**:1107–1111

# 6 When is anal reconstruction required for incontinence and what are the options?

*Constantinos Mavrantonis and Steven D Wexner*

## SURGICAL THERAPY

A number of surgical procedures are available for the treatment of anal incontinence (Table 6.1). The two main methods of surgical treatment are direct repair of an isolated sphincter defect, and reinforcement to supplement the existing sphincter mechanism. A detailed clinical history, physiologic evaluation, and endoanal ultrasonography determine which operation is the most appropriate. In general, available operative techniques attempt to restore the sphincter mechanism, the anorectal angle, or both.

Direct apposition of obstetric sphincter lacerations is usually performed at the time of injury. While results are satisfactory when good technique is adopted, faulty technique, hematoma, wound infection, tension, and unrecognized concomitant sphincter injuries are associated with poor outcome, requiring a secondary repair in at least 0.3–5% or more of patients.[1–3] Patients with isolated sphincter injury not associated with pudendal neuropathy have a better chance of successful outcome following delayed sphincter repair; conversely, multifocal sphincter defects and pudendal neuropathy augur for a poor outcome.[4] Traditionally, for patients in whom all other treatment had failed or was not expected to be efficacious, the only remaining option was a permanent colostomy. However, more recently complex surgical procedures such as implantation or creation of a neosphincter may be an option. Patients presenting with severe traumatic lesions, associated pelvic injuries, and perianal sepsis, are often initially managed with local debridement and a diverting colostomy. Secondary repair is performed after all contaminated perineal wounds have healed and the inflammation has completely subsided.

**Table 6.1** Surgical therapy for fecal incontinence

I  Sphincter repair

   A. Direct apposition

   B. Overlapping repair

      1. External sphincter only

      2. Combined with internal sphincter imbrication

   C. Plication or reefing

      1. Anterior

      2. Posterior

         a. Postanal repair

         b. Puborectalis repair

      3. Total pelvic floor

   D. Thiersch procedure

II  Dynamic neosphincter procedure

   A. Synthetic material

      1. Artificial bowel sphincter

   B. Muscle transfer

      1. Skeletal muscle flaps

         a. Gracilis

            i. stimulated gracilis

         b. Gluteus

         c. Other

      2. Free muscle transplants

III  Diversion

   A. Colostomy

   B. Ileostomy

   C. Continent colonic conduit

# Perineorrhaphy

In conjunction with vaginal colporrhaphy, plication of the perineal body is occasionally performed.[5] The rectovaginal septum is dissected, the excess vaginal mucosa is excised, and the transverse perineal musculature is approximated to reconstruct or reinforce the perineal body. Additional injuries of the anal sphincter must be recognized and repaired.

## Sphincter repair

This procedure is considered for patients with an isolated sphincter defect, as the remaining muscle usually maintains the ability to contract. There are three approaches to sphincter repair: apposition, overlapping, and plication.

### Direct apposition

In 1882 Warren[6] described a perineal repair for sphincter laceration. In 1940, Blaisdell[7] reported the collective results of direct apposition sphincter repair. This technique involves mobilization of the external anal sphincter, division of the muscle, and excision of any scar tissue present. The sphincter is then sutured in an end-to-end fashion. The success rate of this procedure is reported to be between 33 and 77.5%.[8] Failure of this technique has been mainly attributed to separation of the sutured ends of the muscle.

### Overlapping anterior sphincteroplasty

Incontinent patients with an anteriorly disrupted yet functional external anal sphincter muscle are offered overlapping sphincteroplasty as the operation of choice. This procedure, initially described by Parks & McPartlin[9] in 1971 and later modified by Slade *et al.*,[10] has produced better results than has direct apposition and accordingly has gained wider acceptance. It has the advantages of restoration of normal anatomy and function combined with a low incidence of perineal infection.

Preoperative management includes full mechanical bowel preparation using 45 ml sodium phosphate solution twice the day before surgery and intravenous broad-spectrum antibiotics.[11–14] Under general endotracheal or regional anesthesia, patients are placed in the prone jackknife position on a Kraske roll. After sterile preparation of the perianal area, vagina, and perineum, a bilateral nerve block is attained with a mixture of equal parts of 0.5% Xylocaine, 0.25% bupivacaine, and 1:400000 units of epinephrine. A 120 degrees anterolateral incision is made approximately 0.5 cm caudal and parallel to the outer edge of the anal verge, allowing dissection and mobilization of sphincter muscles and scar. In females Anterior dissection is performed with the surgeon's contralateral (nondominant) index finger in the vagina, enabling assessment of tissue thickness and prevention of vaginal wall injury. Lateral dissection where muscle anatomy is usually unaltered can help orientation to the proper plane of dissection. Care is taken to preserve the pudendal nerve bundles that enter the muscles bilaterally, in the posterolateral positions. Mobilization continues from

disappointing results in most adult patients. Salmons & Vroba[61] later demonstrated that type II muscle fibers can be converted to fatigue-resistant slow twitch (type I) fibers, by chronic low-frequency electrical stimulation. Applying this principle to Pickrell's operation, Williams et al.[62] and Baeten et al.[63] each contributed to perfecting this operation. Dynamic graciloplasty may be indicated in selected patients with severe fecal incontinence, where standard therapy has failed or is not expected to be efficacious. Patients must have a rectum, anal canal, and sphincter *in situ* with only partial anatomic defect. Current protocol-mandated contraindications are age under 18 or over 80 years, non-functioning gracilis muscle, cancer of the anorectum or colon, anal agenesis, chronic intractable diarrhea, inflammatory bowel disease, and pregnancy.

The procedure is often performed in two stages. Patients receive mechanical bowel preparation and intravenous and oral antibiotics following the same protocol used for colonic surgery. In the first stage, under general anesthesia without muscular relaxation, the patient is placed in the lithotomy position, with stirrups and a bladder catheter. Both legs are prepped and draped; three incisions in the leg are performed to allow mobilization of the gracilis distally to its insertion onto the tibial tuberosity. While dissecting the proximal neurovascular pedicle, care is taken to avoid skeletonization. Two bilateral radial perianal incisions that communicate through a tunnel around the anus are performed 2 cm from the anal verge. A second tunnel leading from the perineum to the incision in the leg is created, through which the muscle is passed and wrapped around the anus. The tendon is then fixed to the contralateral ischial tuberosity with heavy nonabsorbable sutures. The transposition can be performed using basically three wrap configurations: 'alpha', 'gamma', or 'epsilon'. Regardless of configuration, the muscle rather than the tendon has to be wrapped in a deep rather than a superficial fashion to effect a 'snug' rather than a 'tight' anal closure. Two suction drains are placed in the leg; a stoma is not created.[64]

After a 6- to 9-week period during which the tendon anchors securely to the ischial tuberosity, implantation of the stimulator is undertaken. The technique described by Williams et al.[62] involves direct stimulation of the branch of the obturator nerve by fixing the electrode on the main trunk of the nerve, while Baeten et al. implant the neurostimulator leads inside the muscle, as close as possible to the nerve branches.[65] Direct nerve stimulation theoretically recruits all motor units resulting in high anal pressure. The aim of stimulation however is to obtain continence; maximum contraction may not be necessary for closure of the anal canal.

In a recent study we compared the two techniques of stimulation.[66] Twelve of 13 patients who received intramuscular stimulation had a significantly improved incontinence score; this result has been sustained during a mean follow-up period of $21 \pm 7.4$ months. Conversely, after a mean follow up of $12.5 \pm 7.6$ months, only one of 10 patients who received direct nerve stimulation had shown improvement in continence, although in the early postoperative period a transient improvement was noted in 60% of patients.[67] The cause of treatment failure in these patients was mostly lead migration or lead fibrosis, which resulted in cessation of stimulation due to the small contact surface between the lead and the nerve and the consequent increased impedance.

For the second stage of the operation, patients are prepared as described for the first stage, and the upper incision in the thigh is reopened. In the proximity of the neurovascular pedicle, the site of the maximum muscle contraction is assessed with an external nerve stimulator, and the two intramuscular electrodes are implanted. The electrodes are then tunneled to the lower abdomen where an implantable stimulator is placed in a subcutaneous pocket.

Three days after implantation, a stimulation training protocol of the gracilis muscle wrap is initiated. This protocol consists of progressively reprogramming the stimulator's cycling mode output by increasing the 'on' time and decreasing the 'off' time over an 8-week period. The stimulator is then reprogrammed to the mode for continuous output.

With an external magnet, the patient can switch the neurostimulator on (causing the transposed gracilis muscle to contract) and off (causing the muscle to relax). Patients' ages at surgery did not correlate with the degree of postoperative improvement in continence scores, nor did the duration of the patients' symptoms or body habitus.[66] Etiology of incontinence did not influence outcome nor did the severity of preoperative incontinence, as assessed by incontinence score. Moreover, a history of previous surgery for anal incontinence, early postoperative morbidity, or any of the data obtained from the physiologic investigation (manometric pressures, endoanal ultrasonography and electromyography, and pudendal nerve terminal motor latency findings) were not factors predictive of outcome. Similarly, differences between the preoperative resting and squeeze pressures and the stimulated resting and squeeze pressures 6 months after surgery were not factors predictive of outcome. The issue is raised that anal pressure may not be an adequate indicator of the success of the procedure. In fact, although anal manometry may be relatively insensitive as a predictor of outcome, at the moment it appears to be the best test to quantify muscle function. Clearly, a more accurate tool needs to be developed, which should have better correlation with clinical outcome.

Rongen and Baeten[64] found that patients with incontinence resulting from trauma had a better outcome (92%; $n=24$) than patients with pudendal nerve lesions (64%; $n=14$), caudal lesions (50%; $n=2$), or anal atresia (50%; $n=12$).

In our study,[66] 64% of patients presented with minor or severe complications, such as rupture of tendon, perineal infection, tendon erosion, deep vein thrombosis, anal stenosis, difficult evacuation, fecal impaction, rectal pain, lead infection, fracture of leads, electrode displacement, and electrode fibrosis; most complications were however treatable.

In the series of 52 patients with stimulated graciloplasty published by Baeten and colleagues,[68] 73% continence to solid and liquid stool, after a follow-up period of 2.1 years, was reported. These patients also presented significant improvement in the quality of life assessed by the Nottingham Health Profile[69] and the State-Trait Anger Expression inventory.[70] The mean evacuation frequency had been five per day before transposition, but significantly decreased to two per day 8 weeks after surgery. The median time to defer evacuation increased from 9 seconds prior to stimulation to 19 minutes in 52 weeks, and the mean enema retention time increased from 0 seconds prior to transposition to 3 minutes after 52 weeks. Subsequently, Geerdes and colleagues from the same center[71] reported the results of 67 patients who underwent dynamic graciloplasty. The success rate had reached 78%. Failures were attributed to rectal sensory or distension problems, poor neosphincter contraction, sepsis, and perforation. Eighteen per cent of patients with postoperative 'moderate' constipation were successfully treated with biofeedback and laxatives. This study also reported a high number of complications; however, most complications were either preventable or treatable. A number of patients needed exchange of leads because of infection, tendon shortening for loose wrap, stimulator replacement, and repositioning for displacement. As reported by Korsgen and Keighley,[72] poor rectal sensation augurs for poor results. These patients may experience incomplete evacuation necessitating routine periodic enema washouts.

Mander and colleagues[73] reported their experience with electrically stimulated gracilis neosphincter, following abdominal perineal excision of the rectum, in 12 patients. The underlying disease was adenocarcinoma in 10, anal malignant melanoma in one, and a sweat gland tumor in the other; in all patients, a sphincter-saving resection was contraindicated. In eight patients, the stoma was closed. Median basal and maximum neosphincter pressures were 30 and 122 $cmH_2O$ (294 and 1196 Pa), respectively, in the immediate postoperative period and 22.5 and 76 $cmH_2O$ (220 and 745 Pa), respectively, after 1 year of follow up. All patients whose stomas were closed experienced episodes of incontinence to solid stool and wore pads for persistent fecal soiling. Furthermore, they all reported difficulty in evacuation. Despite imperfect continence, all patients preferred their present status to life with a stoma. Lubowski and colleagues[74] reported a series of 12 patients, five of whom had had an abdominoperineal resection; this subgroup of patients did not benefit as much from the procedure however. As in most series, infection was a prominent early complication.

Results from a modification of stimulated graciloplasty were published by Rosen *et al.*,[75] in which sphincter restoration was performed using one gracilis muscle wrapped around the anus by the 'split sling-technique'. Twenty-seven patients underwent this procedure, with 66% achieving continence for soft and solid stool. The preliminary results of a prospective multicenter trial using the electrically stimulated gracilis neosphincter demonstrated a significant improvement in incontinence scores following stoma closure in 44 out of 51 patients studied.[76]

As an alternative to dynamic graciloplasty, Kumar and colleagues[77] reported good results with bilateral nonstimulated graciloplasty in a series of 10 patients. These patients were followed for a mean of 24 (range 6–40) months, after which nine of the 10 patients were continent. The mean preoperative resting pressure was 16 $cmH_2O$ (157 Pa), whereas postoperatively it significantly increased to 78 $cmH_2O$ (765 Pa). Similarly, the squeeze pressure increased from 44 to 121 $cmH_2O$ (431–1186 Pa), and the high-pressure zone increased from 1 to 2 cm in length.

Dynamic graciloplasty is a relatively safe and reliable technique in selected patients with severe incontinence and may result in a better quality of life. Although the rate of postoperative complications is high, the majority are not life threatening and usually resolve with time and proper management. Patients must have the psychologic strength, emotional commitment, and financial resources, as they may have to go through multiple revisional surgeries. The most important

**Table 6.6** Gracilis transposition

| Author | Year | Patients (no.) | Successful outcome (%) | Infection |
|--------|------|----------------|------------------------|-----------|
| Pickrell et al.*[60] | 1952 | 34 | 100 | — |
| Salmons & Vroba*[61] | 1981 | — | — | — |
| Williams et al.[62] | 1991 | 6 | 0 | — |
| Baeten et al.[63] | 1988 | — | — | — |
| Cavina et al.[78] | 1987 | — | — | — |
| Konsten et al.[79] | 1993 | — | — | — |
| Seccia et al.[80] | 1994 | 75 | 71 | — |
| Baeten et al.[68] | 1995 | 52 | 73 | — |
| Korsgen & Keighley[72] | 1995 | — | — | — |
| Kumar et al.[77] | 1995 | — | — | — |
| Wexner et al.[67] | 1996 | 17 | 60 | — |
| Altomare et al.[81] | 1996 | — | — | — |
| Lubowski et al.[74] | 1996 | — | — | — |
| Geerdes et al.[71] | 1996 | 67 | 78 | 12 |
| Mander & Williams[82] | 1996 | — | — | — |

*Nonstimulated.

variable in a successful outcome following any of the neosphincter procedures is appropriate patient selection. Such procedures certainly needs to be validated through larger series, and modifications are necessary to achieve perfect continence. Initial results however seem promising for those incontinent patients who prefer life without a permanent stoma (Table 6.6).

**Free muscle transplantation.** For the treatment of severe incontinence resulting from congenital absence or traumatic injury to the puborectalis muscle, Hakelius and Olsen[83] proposed a method of free transplantation of the palmaris longus or a segment of the sartorius muscle. This method implies transposition of the palmaris longus, 2 weeks after denervation, to the perirectal area, as a 'U'- sling around the rectum corresponding to the functional position of the puborectalis muscle. After reinnervation of the new muscle has taken place, the muscle becomes part of the reflex mechanism. The authors evaluated the results in 26 totally incontinent children operated on by this method.

After an average of 11 years and 4 months, 60% of the cases were regarded as good, 16% as fair, 8% as improved, and 16% as failures.

**Gluteus maximus transposition.** The gluteus maximus has been the muscle most commonly used for transposition until the 1950s, as initially described by Chetwood in 1902.[84] Patients receive a standard mechanical and oral antibiotic bowel preparation as for elective colorectal surgery, supplemented by perioperative administration of parenteral antibiotics. Regional or general anesthesia may be used and the procedure is performed with the patient in the prone jackknife position with the buttocks taped apart to facilitate exposure. The inferior portion of the origin of each gluteus maximus is detached from the sacrum and coccyx, bifurcated, and tunneled subcutaneously to encircle the anus. The periosteum in each end is then sutured to the ipsilateral split muscle to form two opposing slings of voluntary muscle. In theory, the transposed undivided muscle can distribute the tension of the repair, achieving a closed anus without muscular tension of the neosphincter.[85,86] The transposition of this muscle is facilitated because of its proximity to the anal canal, its thin ventral surface, and its proximal solitary innervation. The gluteus maximus muscle is a large and powerful muscle and its proximity to the perianal area eliminates the need for distant incisions. However, it is a skeletal muscle and cannot assume the function of the internal anal sphincter. This operation is indicated, as are all transposition procedures, in patients with severe neurogenic incontinence, failed previous repairs, and multiple sphincter defects.

There are only a few reported series in the literature and overall the rates of restoration of complete and partial continence are 60 and 36%, respectively. In 1992, Devesa and colleagues[87] published a small series on a modified technique of gluteus maximus transposition for the treatment of traumatic sphincter rupture. The authors performed a unilateral transposition of gluteus maximus in four incontinent patients, with good functional outcomes. The authors stated that although the reported experience with the described technique is limited, the method is easier, seems to have less morbidity than the original technique, and achieves better short-term functional results procured from the thick, tension-free neosphincter. Pearl and coworkers[88] described a nonstimulated bilateral gluteoplasty performed in five men and two women ranging in age from 26 to 65 years. The indications for operation were sphincter destruction secondary to multiple fistulotomies, bilateral pudendal nerve damage, and high imperforate anus with prior surgery. The procedure was performed without the creation of a diverting colostomy. Six out of seven patients became continent to solid stool while only two out of seven were continent to liquids, and only one out of seven continent to flatus. The authors estimated that although resting pressures did not improve, voluntary squeeze pressures were restored and rectal sensation markedly improved. However, these data are somewhat arbitrary, as preoperative and postoperative anal manometry were performed in only four patients. Furthermore, change of equipment during the follow-up period resulted in inaccurate assessment. The patients noted their outcome to be good in four cases, fair in two, and failed in one.

Christiansen and colleagues[89] recently published their results in a series of seven patients, three of whom experienced improved continence after a follow-up period of 1 year, while in four, continence remained unchanged. None of the seven patients, however, rated the operation as 'satisfactory'. Unlike the results reported by Pearl and colleagues,[88] anorectal physiology studies showed moderately increased resting and squeeze pressures in patients who had improved continence.

In 1997, Devesa and colleagues[90] reported the largest series to date, with results not as remarkable as those described by Pearl *et al.*,[88] yet more promising than those of Christiansen *et al.*[89] This study described the clinical experience with adynamic bilateral gluteoplasty in 20 patients with total fecal incontinence, ranging in age from 15 to 58 years, in whom a sphincter repair had failed or was not feasible. The indications for the operation were congenital anomalies, denervation, or sphincter destruction. Morbidity was mostly related to wound infection, requiring reoperations for neosphincter repair, and anal stenosis. Further surgery for tightening of the neosphincter was necessary in two other patients, who ultimately had a successful outcome. Fifty-three per cent of the evaluable patients achieved 'normal' control. Specifically, eight patients were able to retain water instilled into the rectum for between 5 minutes and 2 hours. For patients with improved continence, the mean differences between pre- and postoperative resting and squeeze pressures were 40 and 122 mmHg (356 and 1196 Pa), respectively. Failures were attributed to suture disruption, poor muscular contraction, and intractable constipation. The authors consider adynamic gluteoplasty a more efficient procedure for achieving continence than other adynamic muscle transpositions.

In order to obtain a more pronounced adaptation in the contractile, histochemical, and metabolic properties of muscle fibers, postoperative intermittent long-term stimulation of the gluteus muscle can be performed. Guelinckx and colleagues presented their results in seven patients treated by conventional and four by dynamic gluteoplasty.[91] Patient evaluation revealed continence to stool in nine of the 11 patients; seven of the 11 patients also were continent to liquid stool, including all of the patients who had undergone dynamic gluteoplasties.[91]

It is important to convey to patients an accurate and realistic expectation for a successful outcome with all neosphincter procedures. The satisfactory success rate of these techniques does not imply completely normal continence; some of these patients continue to be incontinent to flatus or are unable to control liquid stool. Furthermore, until they achieve this result, it is possible that they may suffer postoperative complications, the most frequent of which is difficult evacuation. History of preoperative evacuatory impairment or impaired anal sensation has been associated with evacuatory difficulty in recent publications (Table 6.7).

**Table 6.7** Unstimulated bilateral gluteoplasty

| Author | Year | Patients | Results | |
| --- | --- | --- | --- | --- |
| | | | Good | Fair |
| Chetwood[84] | 1902 | 1 | 1 | — |
| Schoemaker[92] | 1909 | 6 | 6 | — |
| Bistrom[93] | 1944 | 3 | 2 | 1 |
| Bruining et al.[94] | 1981 | 1 | 2 | — |
| Prochiantz & Gross[95] | 1982 | 15 | 9 | 1 |
| Hentz[85] | 1982 | 5 | 4 | — |
| Skef et al.[96] | 1983 | 1 | 1 | — |
| Iwai et al.[97] | 1985 | 1 | 1 | — |
| Chen & Zhang[98] | 1987 | 6 | 3 | 1 |
| Onishi et al.[99] | 1989 | 1 | 1 | — |
| Pearl et al.[88] | 1991 | 7 | 4 | 2 |
| Christiansen et al.[89] | 1995 | 7 | 0 | 3 |
| Devesa et al.[87] | 1992 | 10 | 6 | 3 |
| Devesa et al.[90] | 1997 | 17 | 9 | 1 |

**Other muscles.** Other muscles employed for transposition have been the fascia lata, sartorius, and adductor longus. Free muscle transplants utilizing the palmaris longus and the sartorius muscles have also been described, but only in small numbers of patients.

## INDIVIDUALIZING THE APPROACH TO PATIENTS WITH FECAL INCONTINENCE

The wide variety of procedural alternatives is attestation to the lack of universal satisfaction with any single alternative. Part of this dilemma is promulgated by the heterogeneity of the surgical indications, while another contributing factor is the continued deterioration in the quality of results over the last few decades. Recently, it had been hoped that with the more widespread accumulation of anorectal physiologic results predictive criteria could be developed. Sadly, such a prophecy has not been fulfilled. Instead, one must rely upon clinical judgment, historical results, and individual patient's physiologic profile to assign therapeutic terms. Figure 6.1 depicts the Cleveland Clinic Florida's approach to the patient with fecal incontinence.

In general, the patient will present having failed a conservative regimen including diet, antimotility agents, and biofeedback. At that point, physiologic investigation is undertaken including anal manometry, anal ultrasonography, anorectal electromyography with bilateral pudendal nerve terminal motor latency assessment and possibly cinedefecography. If an isolated unifocal (generally anterior) defect is found in a patient with bilaterally normal pudendal nerves, then a multilayered overlapping sphincter repair including puborectalis and intra-anal sphincter imbrication is undertaken. If the pudendal nerves are abnormal and the injury has occurred within the past several months, then conservative management including the anal plug incontinence device and biofeedback would be employed. Hopefully, after additional time has elapsed the pudendal nerves will recover, allowing more reasonable expectations for a successfully overlapping repair after such normalization. Alternatively, if the nerves fail to recover or if the injury has been remote from the time of presentation, then the patient should be informed that, although an overlapping repair is a simple procedure, the chance of success is well under 50%. Furthermore, consideration should be given to one of the neosphincter procedures, rather than forming much anterior scar with a repair that is unlikely to succeed. Not unexpectedly, many

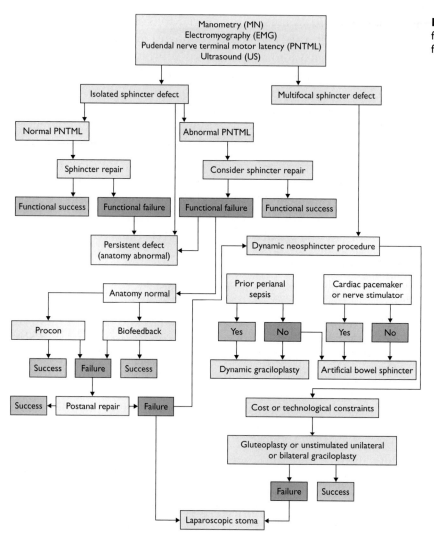

**Fig 6.1** Algorithm for the management of fecal incontinence.

patients are reluctant to undergo a complex procedure until the simpler one has failed. Therefore, although in theory a neosphincter operation would probably confer more satisfactory results in a greater number of patients, in practice, patients with an isolated unifocal defect and bilaterally normal pudendal nerves tend to undergo an overlapping sphincter repair.

If the sphincter repair results in functional failure but repeat physiologic investigation reveals normal anatomy, alternative treatment includes the anal plug incontinence device, biofeedback, or a postanal repair. If, however, a persistent defect is noted on anorectal ultrasonography and/or anorectal electromyography, either a repeat sphincter repair or a neosphincter procedure could be considered.

There are no criteria to determine the appropriateness of either the dynamic graciloplasty or the artificial bowel sphincter. Although specific basic suppositions and caveats may make one procedure more appropriate than the other, if the patient has extensive perineal scarring or significant perianal sepsis, it may be more prudent to transpose well-vascularized muscle than to apply a prosthetic device. Conversely, the implantation of a second electrical device would not be wise in a patient with a pre-existing cardiac pacemaker, implantable defibrillator, or nerve stimulator. In this group, the artificial bowel sphincter is probably preferrable. With these few exceptions, it is difficult to assign patients to one treatment or the other. It is our policy to discuss both procedures with all potential candidates, explaining one is electrical and one is hydraulic. The various risks, benefits, alternatives, and possible complications of each procedure, as well as our group's experience with each operation, is discussed with each patient.

If costs or technological constraints exist, including performance of either the artificial bowel sphincter or the stimulated graciloplasty, then reasonable alternatives for dynamic neosphincter construction include the gluteoplasty, or the unilateral or bilateral unstimulated graciloplasty. These alternatives are suitable in patients with multifocal defects and patients in whom repair of isolated unifocal defects have failed, however, they do not offer the benefit of being under voluntary control.

Ultimately, if the patient fails to gain satisfactory symptomatic relief after this algorithm (Fig. 6.1) has been adopted, then construction of a stoma is a viable option. A well-constructed stoma is more easily managed than is an incontinent and surgically irreparable anus. While it is difficult for many patients to accept this concept, judicious use of enterostomal therapy and group counseling supplemented by literature, illustrations, device samples, and videos can prove very useful. The type of stoma construction would depend upon the patient's history and preference. In general, a left iliac fossa end colostomy would be preferred to an ileostomy of any variety for multiple reasons related to the consistency of stool and the possibility of irrigation. Another option in certain patients is a continent colonic conduit, although this procedure is technically demanding, fraught with the potential for high morbidity, and accordingly not widely employed outside a few centers in the United Kingdom.[100]

## SUMMARY

During the last few decades, sphincter reconstruction and pelvic floor repair have been the established treatment for traumatic and idiopathic fecal incontinence. The results of surgical management of traumatic sphincter defects have been satisfactory, although less impressive in recent years than when initially reported. This deterioration of results is especially pronounced for the postanal procedure. As a result, a number of newer surgical procedures have been devised to treat traumatic or idiopathic fecal incontinence refractory to conventional surgical management. These procedures include transposition of skeletal muscle flaps, primarily the gracilis and gluteus maximus muscles, and the implantation of an artificial anal sphincter. Hopefully, continued analysis of the results of these techniques will allow future generations of patients to be directed to the most appropriate procedure for them. This decision will ideally be based upon preoperative physiologic data and expectation of success with acceptable morbidity. To date, however, this degree of accuracy is not possible.

## REFERENCES

1   Haadem K, Dahlostrom A, Ling L, Ohrlander AS. Anal sphincter function after delivery rupture. *Obstet Gynecol* 1987;**70**:53–70

2   Vencatesh SK, Ramanujam PS, Larson DM, Haywood MA. Anorectal complications of vaginal delivery. *Dis Colon Rectum* 1989;**32**:1039–1041

3   Jacobs PPM, Scheuer M, Kuijpers JHC. Obstetric fecal incontinence: role of pelvic floor denervation and results of delayed sphincter repair. *Dis Colon Rectum* 1990;**33**:494–497

4   Gilliland R, Altomare DF, Moreira H Jr, Oliveria L, Gilliland JE, Wexner SD. Pudendal neuropathy is predictive of failure following anterior overlapping sphincteroplasty. *Dis Colon Rectum* 1998;**41**:1516–1522

5   Nichols DH. Posterior colporrhaphy and perineorrhaphy: separate and distinct operations. *Am J Obstet Gynecol* 1991;**164**:714–721

6   Warren JC. A new method of operation for the relief of rupture of the perineum through the sphincter and rectum. *Trans Am Gynecol Soc* 1882;**7**:324

7   Blaisdell PC. Repair of the incontinent sphincter ani. *Surg Gynecol Obstet* 1940;**70**:692–697

8   Arnaud A, Sarles JC, Sielzneff I, Orsoni P, Joly A. Sphincter repair without overlapping for fecal incontinence. *Dis Colon Rectum* 1991;**34**:744–747

9   Parks AG, McPartlin JF. Later repair of injuries of the anal sphincter. *J R Soc Med* 1971;**64**:1187–1189

10  Slade MS, Goldberg SM, Schottler JL, Balcos EG, Christenson CE. Sphincteroplasty for acquired anal incontinence. *Dis Colon Rectum* 1977;**20**:33–35

11  Cohen S, Wexner SD. Prospective randomized endoscopic-blinded trial comparing precolonoscopy cleansing methods. *Dis Colon Rectum* 1994;**37**:689–696

12  Oliveira L, Wexner SD, Daniel N *et al*. Mechanical bowel preparation for elective colorectal surgery. A prospective, randomized surgeon-blinded trial comparing sodium phosphate and polyethylene glycol-based oral lavage solutions. *Dis Colon Rectum* 1997;**40**:585–591

13  Wexner SD, Beck DE. Sepsis prevention in colorectal surgery. In: Fielding LP, Goldberg SM (eds) *Robb and Smiths Operative Surgery: colon, rectum and anus*, 5th edn. Butterworth-Heinemann, Oxford pp 41–46

14  Vernava AM III, Stratton MD. Preoperative and postoperative management. In: Beck DE, Wexner SD (eds) *Fundamentals of Anorectal Surgery*, 2nd edn. WB Saunders, London, 1998 pp 70–78

15  Wexner SD, Marchetti F, Jagelman DG. The role of sphincteroplasty for fecal incontinence re-evaluated: a prospective physiologic and functional review. *Dis Colon Rectum* 1991;**34**:22–30

16  Ctercteko GC, Fazio VW, Jagelman DG, Lavery IC, Weakley FL, Melia M. Anal sphincter repair: a report of 60 cases and a review of the literature. *Aust NZ J Surg* 1988;**58**:703–710

17  Fleshman JW, Peters WR, Shemesh EI, Fry RD, Kodner IJ. Anal sphincter reconstruction: anterior overlapping muscle repair. *Dis Colon Rectum* 1991;**34**:739–743

18  Browning GG, Motson RW. Anal sphincter injury: management and result of Parks sphincter repair. *Ann Surg* 1984;**199**:351–357

19  Fang DT, Nivatvongs S, Vermeulen FD, Herman FN, Goldberg SM, Rothenberger DA. Overlapping sphincteroplasty for acquired anal incontinence. *Dis Colon Rectum* 1984;**27**:720–722

20  Nessim A, Wexner SD, Agachan F *et al*. Is bowel confinement necessary after anorectal reconstructive surgery?: a prospective randomized trial. *Dis Colon Rectum* 1999;**42**:16–23

21  Laurberg S, Swash M, Henry M. Delayed external sphincter repair for obstetric tear. *Br J Surg* 1988;**75**:786–788

22  Yoshioka K, Keighley MRB. Sphincter repair for fecal incontinence. *Dis Colon Rectum* 1989;**32**:39–42

23  Felt-Bersma RJ, Cuesta MA, Koorevaar M. Anal sphincter repair improves anorectal function and endosonographic image. A prospective clinical study. *Dis Colon Rectum* 1996;**39**:878–885

24  Fleshman JW, Dreznik Z, Fry RD, Kodner IJ. Anal sphincter repair for obstetric injury: manometric evaluation of functional results. *Dis Colon Rectum* 1991;**34**:1061–1067

25  Engel AF, Kamm MA, Sultan AH, Bartram CI, Nicholls RJ. Anterior sphincter repair in patients with obstetric trauma. *Br J Surg* 1994;**81**:1231–1234

26  Engel AF, van Baal SJ, Brummelkamp WH. Late results of postanal repair for idiopathic faecal incontinence. *Eur J Surg* 1994;**160**:637–640

27 Simmang C, Birnbaum EH, Kodner IJ, Fry RD, Fleshman JW. Anal sphincter reconstruction in the elderly; does advancing age affect outcome? *Dis Colon Rectum* 1994;**37**:1065–1069

28 Oliveira L, Pfeifer J, Wexner SD. Physiological and clinical outcome of anterior sphincteroplasty. *Br J Surg* 1996;**83**:502–505

29 Sangwan YP, Coller JA, Barrett RC *et al*. Unilateral pudendal neuropathy. Impact on outcome of anal sphincter repair. *Dis Colon Rectum* 1996;**39**:686–689

30 Sitzler PJ, Thomson JP. Overlap repair of damaged anal sphincter. A single surgeon's series. *Dis Colon Rectum* 1996;**39**:1356–1360

31 Young CJ, Mathur MN, Eyers AA, Solomon MJ. Successful overlapping anal sphincter repair: relationship to patient age, neuropathy, and colostomy formation. *Dis Colon Rectum* 1998;**41**:344–349

32 Londono-Schimmer EE, Garcia-Duperly R, Nicholls RJ *et al*. Overlapping anal sphincter repair for faecal incontinence due to sphincter trauma: five year follow-up functional results. *Int J Colorectal Dis* 1994;**37**:110–113

33 Nikiteas N, Korsgen S, Kumar D, Keighley MRB. Audit of sphincter repair. Factors associated by poor outcome. *Dis Colon Rectum* 1996;**10**:1164–1169

34 Gilliland R, Heymen S, Vickers D, Wexner SD. Biofeedback in the treatment of fecal incontinence. *Br J Surg* 1997;**12**:183(abstract)

35 Mavrantonis C, Wexner SD, Billotti VL, Heymen S, Hamel CT. A new apparatus for treatment of intractable fecal incontinence. *Colorectal Dis* 1999;**1**(suppl 1):42–43 (abstract)

36 Nesselrod JP. *Proctology in General Practice*. WB Saunders, Philadelphia, 1950

37 Parks AG. Anorectal incontinence. *J R Soc Med* 1975;**68**:681–690

38 Parks AG, Porter NH, Hardcastle JD. The syndrome of the descending perineum. *Proc R Soc Med* 1996;**59**:477–482

39 Bartolo DCC, Roe AM, Locke-Edmunds JC. Flap-valve theory of anorectal continence. *Br J Surg* 1986;**73**:1012–1024

40 Womack NR. Morrison JFB, Williams NS. Prospective study of the effects of post anal repair in neurogenic faecal incontinence. *Br J Surg* 1988;**75**:48–52

41 Browning GG, Parks AG. Postanal repair for neuropathic faecal incontinence: correlation of clinical result and anal canal pressures. *Br J Surg* 1983;**70**:101–104

42 Ferguson EF. Puborectalis sphincteroplasty for anal incontinence. *South Med J* 1984;**77**:423–425

43 Habr-Gama A, Alves PA, da Silva e Souza AH, Femenia Viera MJ, Brunetti-Netto C. Treatment of faecal incontinence by post-anal repair. *Coloproctology* 1986;**8**:244–246

44 Scheuer M, Kuijpers HC, Jacobs PP. Postanal repair restores anatomy rather than function. *Dis Colon Rectum* 1989;**32**:960–963

45 Orrom WJ, Miller R, Cornes H, Duthie G, Mortensen NJ, Bartolo DC. Comparison of anterior sphincteroplasty and postanal repair in the treatment of idiopathic fecal incontinence. *Dis Colon Rectum* 1991;**34**:305–310

46 Matsuoka H, Mavrantonis C, Wexner SD *et al*. Postanal repair for fecal incontinence: is it worthwhile? *Dis Colon Rectum* 2000 (in press)

47 Jameson JS, Speakman CT, Darzi A, Chia YW, Henry MM. Audit of postanal repair in the treatment of fecal incontinence. *Dis Colon Rectum* 1994;**37**:369–372

48  Setti-Carraro PS, Kamm MA, Nichols RJ. Long term results of postanal repair for neurogenic faecal incontinence. *Br J Surg* 1994;**81**:140–144

49  Jorge JMN, Wexner SD. Etiology and management of fecal incontinence. *Dis Colon Rectum* 1993;**36**:77–97

50  Keighley MR. Results of surgery in idiopathic faecal incontinence. *S Afr J Surg* 1991;**29**:87–93

51  Pinho M, Ortiz J, Oya M *et al*. Total pelvic floor repair for the treatment of neuropathic fecal incontinence. *Am J Surg* 1992;**163**:340–344

52  Deen KI, Kumar D, Williams JG *et al*. Randomized trial of internal anal sphincter plication with pelvic floor repair for neuropathic fecal incontinence. *Dis Colon Rectum* 1995;**38**:14–18

53  Deen KI, Oya M, Ortiz J, Keighley MR. Randomized trial comparing three forms of pelvic floor repair for neuropathic faecal incontinence. *Br J Surg* 1993;**80**:794–798

54  Christiansen J, Lorentzen M. Implantation of artificial sphincter for anal incontinence. *Lancet* 1987;**2(8553)**:244–245

55  Christiansen J, Lorentzen M. Implantation of artificial sphincter for anal incontinence: report of five cases. *Dis Colon Rectum* 1989;**32**:432–436

56  Christiansen J, Sparso B. Treatment of anal incontinence by implantable prosthetic anal sphincter. *Ann Surg* 1992;**215**:383–386

57  Lehur PA, Michot F, Denis P *et al*. Results of artificial sphincter in severe anal incontinence. Report of 14 consecutive implantations. *Dis Colon Rectum* 1996;**39**:1352–1355

58  Lehur PA, Glemain P, Bruley des Varannes S, Buzelin JM, Leborgne J. Outcome of patients with an implanted artificial anal sphincter for severe faecal incontinence. A single institution report. *Int J Colorectal Dis* 1998;**13**:88–92

59  Wong WD, Jensen LL, Bartolo DC, Rothenberger DA. Artificial anal sphincter. *Dis Colon Rectum* 1996;**39**:1345–1351

60  Pickrell KL, Broadbent R, Masters FW, Metzger JT. Construction of a rectal sphincter and restoration of anal continence by transplanting the gracilis muscle; a report of 4 cases in children. *Ann Surg* 1952;**135**:853–862

61  Salmons S, Vroba G. The influence of activity on some contractile characteristics of mammalian fast and slow muscles. *J Physiol (Lond)* 1967;**192**:39–40

62  Williams NS, Patel J, George BD, Hallan RI, Watkins ES. Development of an electrically stimulated neoanal sphincter. *Lancet* 1991;**9**:338:1166–1169

63  Baeten C, Spaans MD, Fluks A. An implanted neuromuscular stimulator for fecal incontinence following previously implanted gracilis muscle. *Dis Colon Rectum* 1988;**31**:134–137

64  Rongen MJGM, Baeten CGMI. Treatment of fecal incontinence by means of dynamic graciloplasty. *Semin Colon Rectal Surg* 1997;**8**:110–115

65  Baeten CGM, Konsten J, Spaans F *et al*. Dynamic graciloplasty for treatment of faecal incontinence. *Lancet* 1991;**338**:1163–1165

66  Mavrantonis C, Billotti V, Wexner SD. Stimulated graciloplasty for the treatment of intractable fecal incontinence – critical influence of the method of stimulation. *Dis Colon Rectum* 1999;**42**:497–504

67  Wexner SD, Gonzales AP, Rius J, Teoh TA *et al.* Stimulated gracilis neosphincter operation. Initial experience, pitfalls and complications. *Dis Colon Rectum* 1996;**39**:957–964

68  Baeten CGMI, Geerdes BP, Adang EMM *et al.* Anal dynamic graciloplasty in the treatment of intractable fecal incontinence. *N Engl J Med* 1995;**332**:1600–1605

69  Hunt SM, McEwen J, McKenna SP. Measuring health status: a new tool for clinicians and epidemiologists. *J R Coll Gen Pract* 1985;**35**:185–188

70  Forgays DG, Forgays DK, Spielberger CD. Factor structure of the State-Trait Anger Expression Inventory. *J Pers Assess* 1997;**69**:497–507

71  Geerdes BP, Heineman E, Konsten J *et al.* Dynamic graciloplasty. Complications and management. *Dis Colon Rectum* 1996;**39**:912–917

72  Korsgen S, Keighley MRB. Stimulated gracilis neosphincter – not as good as previously thought. Report of four cases. *Dis Colon Rectum* 1995;**38**:1331–1333

73  Mander BJ, Wexner SD, Williams NS *et al.* Preliminary results of a multicentre trial of the electrically stimulated gracilis neoanal sphincter. *Br J Surg* 1999;**86**:1543–1548

74  Lubowski DZ, Kennedy H, Nguyen H. Clinical outcome of stimulated gracilis neosphincter. *Int J Colorectal Dis* 1996;**11**:134(abstract)

75  Rosen HR, Feil W, Novi G *et al.* The electrically stimulated (dynamic) graciloplasty for faecal incontinence first experience with a modified muscle sling. *Int J Colorectal Dis* 1994;**9**:184–186

76  Mander J, Abercombie JF, George B, Williams NS. The electrically stimulated gracilis neoanal sphincter in total anorectal reconstruction. *Int J Colorectal Dis* 1996;**11**:155(abstract)

77  Kumar D, Hutchinson R, Grant E. Bilateral gracilis neosphincter construction for treatment of faecal incontinence. *Br J Surg* 1995;**82**:1645–1647

78  Cavina E, Seccia M, Evangelista G *et al.* Construction of a continent perineal colostomy by using electrostimulated gracilis muscles after abdominoperineal resection: personal technique and experiences with 32 cases. *Ital Surg Sci* 1987;**17**:305–314

79  Konsten J, Baeten CG, Spaans F *et al.* Follow up of anal dynamic graciloplasty for fecal incontinence. *World J Surg* 1993;**17**:404–408

80  Seccia M, Menconi C, Balestri R, Cavina E. Study protocols and functional results in 86 electrostimulated gracilopasties. *Dis Colon Rectum* 1994;**37**:897–904

81  Altomare DF, Rinalde M, Pannakale O, Mimeo V. Electrostimulated gracilis neosphincter: light and shadow of a new procedure. *Int J Colorectal Dis* 1996;**11**:55(abstract)

82  Mander BJ, Williams NS. Patient selection is integral to the success of the electrically stimulated gracilis neosphincter. *Dis Colon Rectum* 1996;**39**:712–713

83  Hakelius L, Olsen L. Free autologous muscle transplantation in children. *Eur J Pediatr Surg* 1991;**1**:353–357

84  Chetwood CH. Plastic operation of the sphincter ani with report of a case. *Med Rec* 1902;**61**:529

85  Hentz VR. Construction of a rectal sphincter using the origin of the gluteus maximus muscle. *Plast Reconstr Surg* 1982;**70**:82–85

86  Girsch W, Rab M, Mader N *et al.* Considerations on stimulated and neosphincter formation: an anatomic investigation in search of alternatives to the gracilis muscle. *Plast Reconstr Surg* 1998;**101**:889–895; discussion 896–898

87  Devesa JM, Vicente E, Enriquez JM *et al.* Total fecal incontinence – a new method of gluteus maximus transposition: preliminary results and report of previous experience with similar procedures. *Dis Colon Rectum* 1992;**35**:339–349

88  Pearl RK, Prasad ML, Nelson RL, Orsay CP, Abcarian H. Bilateral gluteus maximus transposition for anal incontinence. *Dis Colon Rectum* 1991;**34**:478–481

89  Christiansen J, Hansen CR, Rasmussen O. Bilateral gluteus maximus transposition for anal incontinence. *Br J Surg* 1995;**82**:903–905

90  Devesa JM, Fernandez Madrid JM, Rodriguez Gallego B *et al.* Bilateral gluteoplasty for fecal incontinence. *Dis Colon Rectum* 1997;**40**:883–888

91  Guelinckx PJ, Sinsel NK, Gruwez JA. Anal sphincter reconstruction with the gluteus maximus muscle: anatomic and physiologic considerations concerning conventional and dynamic gluteoplasty. *Plast Reconstr Surg* 1996;**98**:293–302

92  Schoemaker J. Un nouveau procede operatoire pour la reconstitution du sphincter anal. *Semin Med* 1909;**29**:160

93  Bistrom O. Plastichesarzatz des M. sphincter ani. *Acta Chir Scand* 1944;**90**:431–438

94  Bruining HA, Bos KE, Colthoff EG *et al.* Creation of an anal sphincter mechanism by bilateral proximally based gluteal muscle transposition. *Plast Reconstr Surg* 1981;**67**:70–73

95  Prochiantz A, Gross P. Gluteal myoplasty for sphincter replacement: principles, results and prospects. *J Pediatr Surg* 1982;**17**:25–30

96  Skef Z, Radhakrishwan J, Reyes HM. Anorectal continence following sphincter reconstruction utilizing the gluteus maximus muscle: a case report. *J Pediatr Surg* 1983;**18**:779–781

97  Iwai N, Kameda H, Tsuto T *et al.* Objective assessment of anorectal function after sphincter reconstruction using the gluteus maximus muscle: report of a case. *Dis Colon Rectum* 1985;**28**:973–977

98  Chen YL, Zhang XH. Reconstruction of rectal sphincter by transposition of gluteus muscle for fecal incontinence. *J Pediatr Surg* 1987;**22**:62–64

99  Onishi K, Maruyama Y, Shiba T. A wrap around procedure using the gluteus maximus muscle for the functional construction of the sphincter in a case of anal incontinence. *Acta Chir Plast* 1989;**31**:56–63

100 Hughes SF, Williams NS. Continent colonic conduit for the treatment of faecal incontinence associated with disordered defecation. *Br J Surg* 1995;**82**:1318–1320

# 7 What is the role of medical treatment in perianal sepsis and fistulas in Crohn's disease?

*James M Church*

## INTRODUCTION

Perianal sepsis occurs in 20–80% of patients with Crohn's disease, and is most often a problem in patients with primary Crohn's proctocolitis. Its presentation varies from mild, relatively asymptomatic anal stenosis to severe sepsis that demands urgent fecal diversion. Its manifestations include fistulas, fissures, abscesses, edematous tags, and ulcers. Patients complain of discharge, pain, bleeding, incontinence, and difficult or incomplete evacuation. When severe, these symptoms can be extremely disabling. Symptoms tend to be worse if there is active proximal disease, which may be in part due to the diarrhea caused by the proximal disease. Even without sepsis a mild to moderate anal stenosis may result from chronic diarrhea.

Complete healing is the ultimate goal in the treatment of perianal Crohn's disease, but patients often accept the lesser outcome of symptomatic improvement. Optimal treatment is both surgical and medical. The roles of medical treatment are to address proximal disease, control stool frequency, and deal with the local presentation. Evaluation of methods of medical treatment is difficult as there have been few randomized studies and because various surgical options are usually performed in addition to medical treatment. In this chapter the different medical options in the treatment of perianal Crohn's disease will be described, along with evidence of their effectiveness. The place of medical therapy in the overall management of patients with perianal Crohn's disease will then be discussed.

## GENERAL CONSIDERATIONS

The first step in managing perianal Crohn's disease is to assess the state of the anus and to drain any suppuration. If the anus cannot be accurately assessed in the office, examination under anesthesia (EUA) is necessary. During the procedure, setons can be placed into any fistulas and tube drains into abscesses. Once the acute presentation is controlled, the next step is to determine the presence and degree of activity of proximal disease. This assessment can be done in part by colonoscopy performed during EUA. Proximal disease is then appropriately treated. Medical treatment instituted for Crohn's enteritis or colitis may help perianal disease, either directly or indirectly. If proximal disease needs surgery, the perianal disease may be a factor in surgical planning. Perhaps a fistula repair can be combined with a resection; possibly, a diverting stoma will help both intra-abdominal and perianal disease.

Once proximal disease is under treatment, medical therapy specific for the perianal disease can be considered. There are four categories of medical treatment: supportive therapy, antibiotics, immunosuppressive therapy, and other treatments.

## SUPPORTIVE THERAPY

Perianal Crohn's disease seems to run a better course if proximal disease, whether in the small bowel or the colon, is treated.[1] Systemic medical treatment has a role in controlling proximal disease and steroids and immunosuppressives used in this way may also influence perianal disease. In patients with chronic diarrhea, use of loperamide, diphenoxylate, or codeine is important to minimize the number of times the anus is used and cleaned per day. Bulk-forming agents will absorb liquid stool and help prevent its leakage onto the perianal skin with subsequent excoriation and worsening of the situation. Gentle anal cleansing with a hand-held shower head, wet towels, or a wet face cloth is encouraged, along with the use of gentle patting or a hair dryer (set on 'cold') for drying. Dressings are frequently changed so that secretions, stool, and mucus are not in prolonged contact with the perianal skin. Elemental diets may offer temporary relief but not permanent healing,[2] while parenteral nutrition has no role as a primary treatment of perianal Crohn's disease.

## ANTIBIOTICS

Metronidazole (250–500 mg three times daily) and ciprofloxacin (500 mg twice daily) are particularly effective in minimizing perianal swelling, edema, and inflammation. They reduce pain and discharge, and some studies report healing of fistulas with metronidazole alone.[3,4] However, metronidazole has side effects that limit its long-term use. Unpleasant taste, persistent nausea and anorexia and an antabuse-type effect are common, but disappear when the drug is stopped. Peripheral paresthesias develop with accumulating dosage and are an indication to stop treatment. Frizelle *et al.* have reviewed studies reporting the use of metronidazole in perianal Crohn's disease and found that of 85 patients in six studies, 36 healed, 34 were better, and 15 did not improve.[5] Eight of the patients who did not improve had the drug for only 1 month. When treatment was stopped, symptoms worsened in about 70% of patients. Ciprofloxacin is often better tolerated than metronidazole, and is equally effective. It has a similar relapse rate when discontinued.[6] If neither of these antibiotics is tolerated, augmentin (500 mg three times daily) can be effective. Culture of the pus may identify other suitable antibiotics. Metronidazole and/or ciprofloxacin are standard adjuvant treatment for surgery, especially if there is cellulitis. For reconstructive procedures such as flap repair of anal fistulas, antibiotics are given for 7–10 days postoperatively. McKee & Keenan reported 127 patients with perianal Crohn's disease treated over a 5-year period. Metronidazole was used in 32 patients and all but two improved. The improvement was long-lasting in seven and temporary in 22.[7]

## The role of antibiotics

Antibiotics are effective in reducing edema, inflammation, and discharge. They are indicated when there are signs of systemic sepsis such as fever or leucocytosis, when other risk factors are present (e.g. diabetes), or when there is cellulitis in addition to abscess or fistula. Antibiotics are important adjuncts to surgery and can be used long term in patients with chronically nonhealing wounds or persistently recurrent sepsis. They are not an alternative to effective drainage and because of the high relapse rates are not usually long-term cures for perianal fistulas.

## IMMUNE MODULATORS

Steroids are not used specifically for perianal Crohn's disease with sepsis, although anorectal ulceration may respond to topical preparations. Systemic steroids are often used to treat proximal disease however, and the presence of undrained anal sepsis in a patient on high-dose (>20 mg prednisone per day) steroids is a dangerous situation. One of the characteristics of Crohn's-related perianal sepsis is its complexity, with multiple internal and external openings. The decreased capacity for healing and for generating a response to inflammation conferred by steroids may allow perianal disease to progress.

Purine analogs have been used successfully to treat perianal Crohn's disease, although no randomized studies have proven their efficacy. 6-Mercaptopurine (6 MP; Puri-Nethol, Glaxo Wellcome) and azathioprine (AZA; Imuran, Glaxo Wellcome) are being used more commonly to treat Crohn's disease in all locations. As physicians become more familiar with the use of these drugs, apprehension about side effects is likely to diminish. The slow onset of action of 6 MP and AZA is a disadvantage, although Sandborn *et al.* describe an intravenous loading technique with AZA.[8] Using 6 MP in a dose of 1.5 mg/kg, Korelitz & Present[9] and Markowitz *et al.*[10] reported fistula healing rates of 64% at 3 months, 95% and 50% at 6 months, and 67% at 1 year. In the long term, remission was sustained as long as treatment was continued. Relapse rates after stopping the medication were high. In a study of intravenous loading of AZA reported by Sandborn *et al.*, five patients with perineal fistulas were included.[8] Two had watering-can perineal disease, and one of these improved. Two other patients had six perianal fistulas between them: all healed. Two patients had rectovaginal fistulas, one of which healed. O'Brien *et al.* treated 78 patients: with AZA (73 patients), with 6 MP (5), or with both (2). Twenty-four of their patients had perianal disease and 18 of these patients responded.[11] In McKee & Keenan's study of 127 patients with perianal Crohn's disease, 41 were treated with AZA. An improvement in symptoms was noted in 28 (68%), and this was permanent in 16 patients.[7]

Side effects of 6 MP and AZA include infectious complications, pancreatitis, fever, rash, leukopenia, nausea/vomiting, and hepatitis. O'Brien *et al.* stopped treatment in eight of 78 patients because of side effects, stopped AZA but later re-instituted 6 MP in two patients, and tapered treatment temporarily in eight patients.[11]

Cyclosporin A (CsA) has been used in patients with perianal Crohn's disease refractory to treatment with purine analogs.[12–14] Dosages are 4 mg/kg/day intravenously and 8 mg/kg/day orally. Using this regimen, both Hanauer *et al.*[12] and Present *et al.*[14] reported a response in seven of 12 patients treated for an average of 6.2 and 12.2 months respectively, although relapses tended to occur when the drug was stopped or given orally. Side effects are paresthesias, hirsutism, nephrotoxicity, and hypertension. A combination of 6 MP/AZA with CsA may lead to opportunistic infections.

Methotrexate is an antimetabolite that inhibits purine synthesis. Its use in patients with perianal Crohn's disease has been described by Kozarek *et al.*[15] They treated 14 patients with 25 mg/week for 12 weeks and found that symptoms improved in 11. However, improvement took up to 10 weeks to be evident. Side effects of methotrexate include diarrhea, nausea, leukopenia, and hepatotoxicity.

## The role of immune modulators

Immune modulators are an alternative to surgery in trying to achieve healing of chronic perianal wounds and perianal fistulas. In the long term surgery is a better form of treatment however, as the beneficial effect of drugs lasts only for as long as they are given. Before using immune modulators to try and heal perianal Crohn's disease, conventional surgery should be tried, or fistulas and wounds should be surgically optimized. Specifically, abscesses should be drained and allowed to contract, granulation tissue should be curetted, fistulas should be 'simplified', and cellulitis resolved. In circumstances where primary surgical repair is impossible (when the anus and lower rectum are ulcerated so that a flap repair is impossible) or unacceptable (when fecal diversion or proctectomy is recommended), immune modulators assume a primary role. In these situations, long-term treatment with 6 MP or AZA may be acceptable to patient and physician. CsA or methotrexate may be used in the short term to achieve healing in patients resistant to 6 MP or AZA. Once the disease is healed, maintenance 6 MP/AZA may be instituted.

## OTHER APPROACHES

For patients with severe perianal disease in whom conventional medical and surgical approaches have failed, two other treatments are available. One of the latest developments in the medical treatment of patients with

Crohn's disease is the anti-tumor necrosis factor α (TNF-α) chimeric antibody (infliximab (Remicade), Centocor, Inc., Malvern, PA). Early data show a benefit from one infusion in two-thirds of patients with perianal Crohn's disease.[16] The benefit lasted at least 3 months. Infliximab is a potential alternative to repeated, radical, or sphincter-removing surgery in severe cases of perianal Crohn's disease. It is also a less toxic alternative to CsA and methotrexate when attempting to induce remission in severe, nonsurgical disease.

Hyperbaric oxygen therapy has been successfully used in patients with perianal Crohn's disease. Brady *et al.*[17] first showed that this could be effective and Colombel *et al.*[18] treated eight patients with at least 30 sessions each. Three had complete healing and three had partial healing. Lavy *et al.* had even more success in six patients who had failed metronidazole and 6 MP. Four of the six had complete healing and two were significantly improved.[19] The limited availability of this treatment option, however, restricts its use on a routine basis.

## The role of other approaches

The role of infliximab in perianal Crohn's disease has yet to be defined but early results are encouraging. It is unlikely to be a permanent solution but may provide short-term healing in difficult cases where diversion or proctectomy is the only alternative. Hyperbaric oxygen is worth trying when it is available but, as with all other medical treatments, it is unlikely to be a long-term solution.

## SUMMARY

Perianal Crohn's disease is difficult to manage, either medically or surgically. There are two primary goals: to heal the anus and to keep it healed. Both surgical and medical treatment can achieve healing; long-term medical therapy is needed to prevent relapse. The role of medical therapy is as an adjunct to surgery, both in producing an initial resolution of the disease and in maintaining this remission. This sort of unified approach is summarized in the algorithm in Figure 7.1. The types of responses that can be expected are shown in Table 7.1.

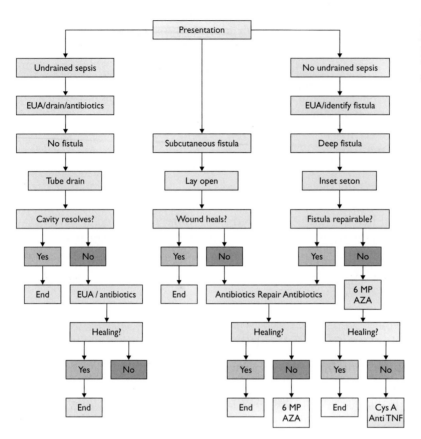

**Fig 7.1** An algorithm for the treatment of patients with perianal Crohn's fistula or sepsis.

**Table 7.1** Reported response rates to medical therapy for perianal Crohn's disease

| Drug | References | Patients (no.) | Duration of treatment | Response |
|---|---|---|---|---|
| Metronidazole | 3, 4, 20 | 74 | 5–35 month | 49% healed<br>42% improved |
| 6 MP | 9, 10 | 68 | 3 month–5 yr | 68% after 6 months<br>78% after 1 year |
| Azathioprine/6 MP | 11 | 24 | | 75% |
| Methotrexate | 15 | 14 | | 79% |
| Cyclosporine A | 12, 13, 14 | 24 | 3–6 month | 75% |
| Infliximab | 16 | 63 (90% perianal fistulas) | 3 infusions/6 wk | 62% partially closed<br>46% completely closed |

# REFERENCES

1    Wolff BG, Culp CE, Beart RW *et al*. Anorectal Crohn's disease; a long term perspective. *Dis Colon Rectum* 1985;**28**:709–711

2    Calam J, Crooks PE, Walker RJ. Elemental diet in the management of Crohn's perianal fistula. *J Parenter Enteral Nutr* 1979;JPEN **4**:4–8

3    Bernstein LH, Frank MS, Brandt LJ, Boley SJ. Healing of perianal Crohn's disease with metronidazole. *Gastroenterology* 1980;**79**:357–365

4    Brandt LJ, Bernstein LH, Boley SJ *et al*. Metronidazole therapy for perineal Crohn's disease: a follow-up study. *Gastroenterology* 1982;**83**:383–387

5    Frizelle FA, Santoro GA, Pemberton JH. The management of perianal Crohn's disease. *Int J Colorectal Dis* 1996;**11**:227–237

6    Turunen U, Farkkila M, Voltonen V *et al*. Long term outcome of ciprofloxacin treatment in severe perianal or fistulous perianal Crohn's disease. *Scand J Gastroenterol* 1989;**24**(suppl):144

7    McKee RF, Keenan RA. Perianal Crohn's disease – is it all bad news? *Dis Colon Rectum* 1996;**39**:136–142

8    Sandborn WJ, Van Os EC, Zins Bjet *et al*. An intravenous loading dose of azathioprine decreases the time to response in patients with Crohn's disease. *Gastroenterology* 1995;**109**:1808–1817

9    Korelitz BI, Present DH. Favorable effect of 6-mercaptopurine on fistulae of Crohn's disease. *Dig Dis Sci* 1985;**30**:58–64

10   Markowitz J, Rosa J, Grancher K *et al*. Long term 6-mercaptopurine treatment in adolescents with Crohn's disease. *Gastroenterology* 1990;**99**:1347–1351

11   O'Brien JJ, Bayless TM, Bayless JA. Use of azathioprine or 6-mercaptopurine in the treatment of Crohn's disease. *Gastroenterology* 1991;**101**:39–46

12   Hanauer SB, Smith MB. Rapid closure of Crohn's fistulas with continuous intravenous cyclosporine A. *Am J Gastroenterol* 1993;**88**:646–649

13   Brynsov J, Freund L, Rasmussen A. A placebo-controlled, double blind randomized trial of cyclosporine therapy in active Crohn's disease. *N Engl J Med* 1989;**321**:845–850

14   Present D, Lichtiger S. Efficacy of cyclosporine in treatment of fistula of Crohn's disease. *Dig Dis Sci* 1994;**39**:374–380

15   Kozarek RA, Patterson DJ, Gelfand MD *et al*. Methotrexate induces clinical and histological remission in patients with refractory inflammatory bowel disease. *Ann Intern Med* 1989;**110**:353–356

16   Present A, Mayer L, VanDeventer SJH *et al*. Anti-TN-alpha chimeric antibody (cA2) is effective in the treatment of the fistulae of Crohn's disease: a multicenter, randomized, double-blind, placebo-controlled study. *Am J Gastroenterol* 1997;**92**:A648 (abstract)

17    Brady CE, Cooley BJ, Davis JC. Healing of severe perianal and cutaneous Crohn's disease with hyperbaric oxygen. *Gastroenterology* 1989;**97**:756–760

18    Colombel JF, Mathieu D, Bouault JM *et al*. Hyperbaric oxygenation in severe perianal Crohn's disease. *Dis Colon Rectum* 1995;**38**:609–614

19    Lavy A, Melamed Y, Weiss G, Eidelan S. Hyperbaric oxygen heals perianal fistulas in Crohn's disease. *Gastroenterology* 1992;**102**:651

# 8 What are the continuing challenges and issues related to restorative proctocolectomy?

*Zane Cohen*

## INTRODUCTION

The pelvic pouch or restorative proctocolectomy has become the procedure of choice for the majority of patients with ulcerative colitis and familial adenomatous polyposis who require surgery. Although the morbidity rate after this operation is somewhat higher than for a standard total proctocolectomy and conventional ileostomy,[1] it has the advantage of restoring gastrointestinal continuity and allowing patients to live a stoma-free existence. The procedure has evolved over the past two decades. However, there are still several issues which are somewhat controversial and further challenges that must be faced.

There is still debate as to the optimal level of the pouch anal anastomosis and whether it should be a stapled or a hand-sewn anastomosis with a mucosectomy. The need for a defunctioning ileostomy has been questioned as it has been suggested that it is more advantageous for the patient to have a single-stage procedure. The cancer risk in leaving a 1–2 cm anal columnar mucosal epithelium is undetermined and surveillance and management of dysplasia, if found in the residual anal rectal cuff or in the pouch itself, are unclear. Pouchitis occurs more commonly in patients with ulcerative colitis than those with familial adenomatous polyposis; its management and the relationship of recurring episodes of pouchitis to the potential development of neoplasia have not been defined. The influence of age on functional results and the outcome in patients with Crohn's disease or indeterminate colitis have also been argued. If there is benefit in the quality of life after restorative proctocolectomy, this should be measured against other forms of surgical management.

These are some of the issues and challenges that are discussed.

## STAPLED ANASTOMOSIS VERSUS HAND-SEWN ANASTOMOSIS AND MUCOSECTOMY

It has been shown that a long rectal cuff is not necessary in order to achieve a good functional result.[2] The present surgical practise is to leave 1–2 cm rectal muscular cuff and to perform either a complete mucosectomy with a hand-sewn ileoanal anastomosis or a stapled ileoanal anastomosis leaving the anal transitional zone as well as 1–2 cm of anal mucosa.[3–5] The factors to be considered are the functional result and the leak rate of a hand-sewn versus a stapled anastomosis and the risk of developing carcinoma in the residual anorectal mucosa when a stapled anastomosis is performed.

There have now been three randomized controlled studies in a small number of patients,[6–8] the first of which was by Seow-Choen, comparing hand-sewn versus stapled anastomosis, which have shown no differences in functional results. However, the vast majority of uncontrolled reports with much larger numbers,[9–13] have demonstrated that the functional results are better with a stapled anastomosis.

The reason for this discrepancy is understandable. In order to perform a mucosectomy with a hand-sewn anastomosis, the anus is often continually dilated. It has been well demonstrated that physiologically the resting anal pressure decreases dramatically following this procedure[14] and requires a significant period of time to return to almost normal levels. Conversely, a large-size stapler may also interfere, at least temporarily, with the anal resting pressure.[15] Accordingly it is recommended that for a stapled anastomosis, a stapler size not larger than 28–29 mm is used. Even if relative narrowing develops at the anastomosis, there is usually no impairment of function because of the looseness of the stool. In stapled anastomosis the retained anal transitional zone has a functional role in anal continence, which may also account for the better result.

In our experience the leak rate significantly decreased with the use of the stapled as opposed to a hand-sewn anastomosis.[15] Similarly, the functional results have also improved.

Concern about dysplasia or cancer developing in the residual columnar mucosa in stapled anastomosis has not been substantiated. At the Cleveland Clinic, after an average follow up of 2–3 years with annual biopsies, eight of 254 patients were found to have low-grade dysplasia in the anal transitional zone but only two had persistent dysplasia with repeat biopsy. They underwent complete mucosectomy with pouch advancement to the dentate line. Neither had any signs of malignancy in the excised mucosa and, interestingly, both had dysplasia in the colectomy specimens.[16] Patients after hand-sewn anastomosis are not exempt from surveillance because they share the risk of developing dysplasia in the pouch. Furthermore, after mucosectomy, 20% of patients will have remnants of columnar epithelium.[17]

Hence, in most cases a stapled ileal anastomosis is regarded as the procedure of choice when performing restorative proctocolectomy for ulcerative colitis. However, a mucosectomy and hand-sewn ileoanal anastomosis should be considered in patients with dysplasia and/or colonic cancer, in those with familial adenomatous polyposis, and in those who have extraintestinal manifestations associated with their disease, including primary sclerosing cholangitis. In these patients, the risk of developing neoplasia in the residual anorectal mucosa may be greater.

## THE DEFUNCTIONING ILEOSTOMY VERSUS MULTI-STAGED PROCEDURE

The increasing experience and confidence in performing restorative proctocolectomy has raised the question of the routine need of a defunctioning ileostomy. In our own series there was a significantly higher anal anastomotic leak rate in those patients in whom a covering loop ileostomy was omitted.[18] However, very few of these patients required reoperation in the form of a defunctioning ileostomy; in 11 of 13 patients, the leaks healed spontaneously with tube drainage and antibiotic therapy. None of the procedures were considered failures, because none of the pouches were removed. Although these patients have functionally done well, an ileoanal anastomotic leak is still the most frequent cause of pouch failure.[19] The incidence of anastomotic disruption with local sepsis after restorative proctocolectomy, even with a defunctioning ileostomy, ranges from 5 to 15% in larger reported series.[20,21]

A number of reports have argued that ileostomy is unnecessary in the majority of patients undergoing restorative proctocolectomy,[22,23] as the complications related to the loop ileostomy and its closure outweigh the risk taken by avoiding it. The reported incidence of stomal complications has varied and has included small-bowel obstruction around the base of the loop ileostomy and, following its closure, high ileostomy output and anastomotic leaks at the site of closure.[22,23] Furthermore, ileoanal anastomotic leaks can become evident after closure of an ileostomy, necessitating yet another operation. Therefore, there is a significant saving in total hospital stay and in operating time in patients who do not have a covering ileostomy.[22,23] This is disputed because although patients may recover uneventfully, some suffer diarrhea and anal excoriation postoperatively, which prolongs their hospital stay.

However, caution should be exercised in recommending the routine omission of an ileostomy. Despite the fact that leaks at the ileoanal anastomosis in patients without a defunctioning ileostomy heal with conservative management, in our overall series a leak at the ileoanal anastomosis is the most significant factor in pouch failure. In nonrandomized series the pelvic sepsis rates are lower in diverted patients than in patients who have a one-staged procedure.

The current controversy therefore regarding whether an ileostomy should be performed involves weighing the risk and morbidity of developing an ileoanal anastomotic leak against the morbidity and increased hospitalization associated with loop ileostomy and its subsequent closure. At present, we would still favor performing a defunctioning loop ileostomy in patients in whom a colectomy and ileoanal pouch anastomosis are synchronously performed and in all patients who have a hand-sewn ileoanal anastomosis with a mucosectomy. Those patients with acute ulcerative colitis who are nutritionally depleted, or on large doses of steroids or cyclosporine, and have lost weight and are anemic, initially require a colectomy and ileostomy. When they have fully recovered and are in a more favorable condition we would then perform abdominal proctectomy and a stapled restorative ileoanal pouch without a covering defunctioning loop ileostomy unless there is intraoperative difficulty with the anastomosis or a mucosectomy with a hand-sewn ileoanal anastomosis is carried out. The ileostomy would be closed approximately 3 months later. This strategy is the safest way to achieve the best possible outcome (Fig. 8.1).

## POUCHITIS, DYSPLASIA, AND CANCER

Pouchitis can be either an acute or a chronic inflammatory condition or both. It occurs in up to 40% of patients with ileal pouches.[24] The exact incidence of pouchitis is unknown because of the lack of

**Fig 8.1** Management methods for patients presenting having had a colectomy and for patients presenting for the first stage of a pelvic pouch.

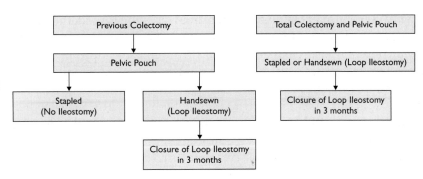

uniformity in its definition in various reports. It is likely to be due to bacterial changes in the luminal content, and it can mimic a human form of inflammatory bowel disease. Other etiologic factors that have been suggested and have been debated are the pouch size, outflow obstruction of the pouch, stasis in the pouch, pouch ischemia, abnormal mucus, insufficient short-chain fatty acids in the pouch, excessive release of inflammatory mediators, and immunologic or hormonal imbalance. I believe that it is a distinct entity, different from that of ulcerative colitis and/or Crohn's disease. All ileal pouches performed as part of restorative proctocolectomy show chronic inflammatory changes. This contrasts distinctly with the findings in ileal pouches that are constructed for continent urinary diversion, where the degree of inflammation is significantly less. Although mild chronic inflammatory changes in ileal pouches of patients who have undergone restorative proctocolectomy for familial adenomatous polyposis are also seen, acute inflammatory changes are relatively rare.

The symptoms of pouchitis include excessive watery stools, often bloody, fatigue, fever, anemia, and, occasionally, weight loss. Endoscopically, it can appear as mild, moderate, or severe. There may be mild changes with some superficial ulceration, which must be distinguished from ulcerations that may occur due to ischemia along the staple line used to construct the ileal pouch. More severe inflammatory changes may even mimic changes seen in a 'typical' case of ulcerative colitis. Pouchitis usually occurs toward the base of the ileal pouch, although it can occur anywhere within the pouch. It is treated with oral antibiotics: the most effective combination is ciprofloxacin (500 mg, twice daily) and metronidazole (250 mg, three times daily) for a minimum period of 2 weeks. The majority of patients will have one attack; however, those with recurrent episodes may have to be maintained on this antibiotic regime for several months. In some cases, small doses of antibiotics will have to be administered on a continual basis as maintenance to minimize symptoms. Patients who fail to respond to this initial therapy may require topical 5-aminosalicylic acid or steroid enemas. Although medical therapy is effective, about 10% of patients regard their pouchitis as a medical, social, and occupational encumbrance when a diversion ileostomy or pouch excision may have to be considered.[25]

Villous atrophy is a consistent histologic change in patients with ileal pouches. However, with chronic episodes of pouchitis, villous atrophy may be severe and, therefore, the risk of dysplasia is greater. In several large series of patients, pouchitis and high-grade dysplasia were rare long-term causes of pouch failure, occurring in only about 2% of patients.[20,26]

To date, five cancers have been reported in the literature associated with restorative proctocolectomy.[27–31] On close review of these cases, three have occurred in the rectal cuff in patients who had undergone restorative proctocolectomy with a mucosectomy for ulcerative colitis in two who interestingly had dysplasia in the colectomy specimens and one patient was operated on for familial adenomatous polyposis. In our own series, one patient with a cuff cancer was reported[27] in our earlier experience when a 10–12 cm rectal cuff was left *in situ* having been stripped of its mucosa. Our present technique is to dissect the rectum to the pelvic floor, leaving only 1–2 cm of residual columnar epithelium. This short area is easier to visualize and gives a maximum degree of confidence that all mucosa is removed when a mucosectomy is performed.

There have been two cases of cancer in the ileal pouch itself performed for ulcerative colitis; one was in a Kock ileal pouch.[30,31] Therefore, the total number of true ileal pouch cancers and of cancers in the residual rectal cuff following a stapled restorative proctocolectomy is extremely low given the total number of pouches performed worldwide. This, although of potential concern, should not give rise to panic. It is, however, important that patients are informed about the small risk of the development of cancer in the ileal pouch where the indication for surgery is ulcerative colitis.

The question of cancer in the ileal pouch itself should not be taken in isolation, as there is also a less than 1% reported incidence of cancer developing at the stomal site of patients who have undergone total proctocolectomy and ileostomy for ulcerative colitis.[32] In addition to those cases of cancer reported in ulcerative colitis, there have been three reported in relation to the ileal pouch of patients who have undergone restorative proctocolectomy for familial adenomatous polyposis. The development of polyps within an ileal pouch in familial adenomatous polyposis patients as precursor lesions to the development of cancer is discussed below.

In summary, there has been a worldwide experience of 30 years with the ileal pouch, including both the Kock and the pelvic pouch. Very few cancers have been reported. Our efforts should focus on those patients at high risk of developing cancer and on recommending a surveillance program.

## SURVEILLANCE AFTER ILEOANAL POUCHES

In 1991, Löfberg *et al.*[33] reported on a patient with an 18-year history of ulcerative colitis who underwent restorative proctocolectomy and was followed by endoscopic biopsy sampling from the pouch at regular intervals. There was gradual development of severe atrophy in the ileal mucosa followed by the development of low-grade dysplasia. Four years after construction of the pouch, biopsies were sampled for flow cytometric DNA analysis. DNA aneuploidy was detected in a biopsy from the center of the pouch and a biopsy taken immediately adjacent showed low-grade dysplasia. In a follow-up report, five patients were found to have low-grade dysplasia with aneuploidy. These patients were enrolled in a surveillance program where biopsies were taken from the top, mid-portion, and base of the pouch. To date, none of these patients have developed cancer or been operated upon.

We have recently studied over 100 patients with longstanding ileal pouches. The group included patients who had recurrent episodes of pouchitis; patients who had not had pouchitis all with an initial diagnosis of ulcerative colitis; patients with an initial diagnosis of familial adenomatous polyposis; and patients with Kock pouches or with incontinent ileostomies after proctocolectomy for ulcerative colitis. All these patients underwent endoscopic examination and multiple biopsies from the top, mid-portion, and base of the pouch as well as from the residual mucosa when present. One of over 800 biopsies taken showed low-grade dysplasia, which was confirmed by two expert gastrointestinal pathologists; this patient had associated aneuploidy found on flow cytometry, but there was no evidence of cancer. There was also no past history of pouchitis. Two other patients had aneuploidy, discovered on flow cytometry, but with no evidence of dysplasia in the biopsy specimens.

What is the correct course of action to be taken in these challenging patients? At present, there is no correct answer. The one patient who had a biopsy with low-grade dysplasia was informed of the uncertainty about the true risk of progression to severe dysplasia and/or cancer. This particular patient could not psychologically live with the fact that a cancer might be present or subsequently develop and opted to have the pouch excised. The initial pathology report showed no evidence of dysplasia; however, after an additional 130 sections were taken one revealed a low-grade dysplasia.

This case exemplifies the dimension of the challenge that we are facing. Irrespective of the enormity of surveillance and tissue sampling, one can never be absolutely certain that dysplasia and the development of cancer can be confidently ruled out. It is likely that many patients with longstanding ileal pouches have low-grade dysplasia that will remain undetected and, therefore, its significance will remain unknown.

Despite the above admonitions, we must make every effort to maximize the detection of dysplasia in order to minimize the occurrence of cancer. In order to achieve this, the International Organization of Inflammatory Bowel Disease (IOIBD) will be making recommendations for surveillance and follow up which are likely to be similar to those recommendations made for long-term patients with chronic ulcerative colitis. In those patients who have had a functioning restorative proctocolectomy for more than 8–10 years, periodic endoscopic visualization of the pouch with multiple random biopsies should be performed. In those patients who are symptomatic with episodes of pouchitis, endoscopic and histologic confirmation of pouchitis should be obtained. In addition, for those patients who have had restorative proctocolectomy with a stapled anastomosis where residual mucosa is left *in situ*, the total length of the disease process should be considered and a surveillance program of the residual mucosa commensurate with the length of the disease process itself instituted. The current recommendation is to follow the residual anorectal mucosa in patients who have had a total history of ulcerative colitis of at least 8–10 years.

A follow up of patients who have restorative proctocolectomy for familial adenomatous polyposis is even more disconcerting. In our own series as well as in at least one other,[34] the recurrence of small polyps in the ileal pouch of patients with familial adenomatous polyposis is in the order of 50–60%. What should be done with these particular patients? The answer again is unknown. These patients may have a genetic mutation on chromosome 5 which predisposes them not only to severe polyposis, but to the development of polyps in the ileal pouch following restorative proctocolectomy. In 18 patients who had undergone restorative proctocolectomy and had developed further polyps, we have not been able to correlate a specific mutation site with the development of polyps in the ileal pouch. However, the numbers are small and efforts to find a genetic association should continue despite the negative findings to date. The use of nonsteroidal anti-inflammatory drugs or of cyclooxygenase inhibitors may be of benefit in the future to these patients.

## INDETERMINATE COLITIS AND CROHN'S COLITIS

Patients enthusiastically endorse the pelvic pouch procedure to avoid a permanent stoma. Even in the early years, when complication rates were high, many patients chose this operation. In recent years with decreased morbidity and failure rate, the pelvic pouch procedure has become the procedure of choice for most patients who require surgery for ulcerative colitis and in selected patients with familial adenomatous polyposis. In cases where an absolute diagnosis cannot be made between ulcerative colitis and Crohn's disease, the patient is usually labeled with the diagnosis of 'indeterminate colitis'. Indeterminate colitis is neither a specific disease nor a new disease. In 10–15% of cases it is impossible for the pathologist and for the clinician to use clinical and pathological criteria to determine the exact disease status.[35] It has been shown in numerous reports that those patients with 'indeterminate colitis' act more like patients with ulcerative colitis following restorative proctocolectomy than individuals with Crohn's disease.[36] The main difference seen was in the long-term failure rate, which was 19% in the indeterminate group and only 8% in the ulcerative colitis group.[37] We still believe that a known diagnosis of Crohn's disease precludes having restorative proctocolectomy. However, recently there have been unpublished reports of patients with longstanding Crohn's colitis who have undergone restorative proctocolectomy with good results. The published literature does not support this conclusion. Patients with prior perianal disease whose quality of life has not been good because of colonic disease as well as perianal disease may still be considered for the pelvic pouch procedure. However, a recent study by our own group has shown that restorative proctocolectomy may be an acceptable surgical alternative for selected patients with prior perianal disease because the overall pouch failure rate is not significantly increased compared with patients without prior perianal disease.[36]

## AGE LIMITATION

We must be cautious about offering this operation to individuals over the age of 50. It has been shown in various reports that the functional outcome is not as good in these patients as it is in patients under the age of 50[38,39] and there is deterioration in overall function between the third to the seventh decades of life at 3 and 12 months after operation in patients undergoing restorative proctocolectomy.[40] We have examined the outcome and surgical complication rate in patients over and under the age of 40 and found that the leak rate at the ileal pouch anastomosis was higher in the older patients and, as observed by others, soiling and the number of stools per day were increased in patients over the age of 50 compared with younger patients. Conversely, Lewis *et al.*[41] found that the resting and maximum squeeze pressures were not different between patients over and under the age of 50, before and after the operation. Mild differences in the incidence of mucus leakage and the ability to discriminate flatus from feces were not significant between the groups. Taking medical fitness in elderly patients into account, the higher morbidity associated with restorative proctocolectomy would favor alternative surgical management, particularly when the quality of life may not be determinately different as discussed later. Furthermore, older patients are less resentful of a permanent stoma with the prospect of safety and symptomatic cure. Therefore, this operation should be offered cautiously and discussed carefully with patients over the age of 50.

## QUALITY OF LIFE

Several studies have attempted to assess patients' quality of life after various procedures[42–44] although not in randomized controlled trials. Therefore, some differences may result because of the patient cohorts studied, and the individual patient's preferences. These deficiencies may limit the relevance of the findings in these studies. In addition, most of the comparative studies have been performed using questionnaires, which are nonvalidated instruments. In one of the largest studies Kohler et al.[45] surveyed 406 patients who underwent conventional ileostomy, 403 who underwent the Kock pouch procedure, and 300 who underwent restorative proctocolectomy for either ulcerative colitis or familial adenomatous polyposis. More than 90% of patients in each of the three groups were satisfied with their current status, although 33% of patients with a conventional ileostomy, 11% of patients with a Kock pouch, and 3% with a pelvic pouch preferred to have a change. More than 90% of the patients in all three groups had returned to normal activity, and more than 60% reported their attitude had improved since surgery.

McLeod et al.[43] used two techniques to assess the quality of life after these procedures: the time trade-off technique and the direct questioning of objectives to derive utilities for patients' perceived health status. A utility of 1.0 signified perfect health. There were 28 patients who underwent conventional ileostomy, 28 who underwent continent ileostomy, and 37 who underwent the pelvic pouch procedure. All of the patients had had surgery at least 1 year previously and were randomly selected. The mean utility values for all of these groups of patients was 0.87–0.97, which approached normality in all three groups. There were no specific differences in these utilities between these groups. The study suggested that quality of life is close to that of 'normal' individuals after any of the three procedures. This study was similar to another study,[44] where quality of life was comparable in one group who underwent total proctocolectomy and ileostomy to that of another group who underwent restorative proctocolectomy. The validated tool used to measure quality of life was the inflammatory bowel disease questionnaire. The level of satisfaction with respect to the procedures was also the same.

These studies, among others, have shown that quality of life is very high in most patients after surgery, irrespective of the procedure performed. The perception of having a stoma of any kind is known to be worse than the reality. This anxiety may account for the reason why most patients elect to have restorative proctocolectomy over other procedures, despite the fact that restorative proctocolectomy has a higher morbidity rate than total proctocolectomy and ileostomy.

The issue of quality of life measurement is difficult. A further challenge to restorative proctocolectomy is to pursue further studies using validated measurements of quality of life to compare the surgical procedures performed. The findings from the above studies should not discourage surgeons from considering the various alternative procedures. Rather, surgery should be viewed as a very effective treatment for patients with ulcerative colitis and patients should play a role in selecting the best procedure, based on their expectations and lifestyle. The challenge for surgeons is to decide on the optimal surgical procedure for each individual patient.

## SUMMARY

This chapter has attempted to highlight not only the controversial issues of restorative proctocolectomy but also the further challenges that all health-care workers face with regard to the longer-term follow up of patients with ileal pouches. It has also challenged surgeons, in particular, to provide the patient with a full understanding of the outcomes and potential complications following restorative proctocolectomy in comparison to other surgical alternatives available. There is no single operation which is always suitable for all patients. Honesty, a detailed informed consent, and the availability of the entire spectrum of surgical options give the best methods of optimizing outcome and ensuring patient satisfaction.

## REFERENCES

1    Wong WD, Rothenberger DA, Goldberg SM. Ileo-anal pouch procedures. *Curr Probl Surg* 1985;**22**:9–77

2    Grant D, Cohen Z, McHughs *et al*. Restorative proctocolectomy: clinical results and manometric findings with long and short rectal cuffs. *Dis Colon Rectum* 1986;**29**:27–32

3    Heald RJ, Allen DR. Stapled ileo-anal anastomosis: a technique to avoid mucosal proctocolectomy in ileal pouch operations. *Br J Surg* 1986;**73**:571–572

4    Dozois RR, Goldberg SM, Rothenberg DA *et al*. Restorative proctocolectomy with ileal reservoir. *Int J Colorectal Dis* 1986;**1**:2–19

5    Williams NS, Marzouk DEMM, Hallan RI, Waldron DJ. Function after ileal pouch and stapled pouch-anal anastomosis for ulcerative colitis. *Br J Surg* 1989; **79**:1168–1171

6    Seow-Cheon F, Tsunoda A, Nicholls RJ. Prospective randomized trial comparing anal function after hand-sewn ileo-anal anastomosis with mucosectomy versus stapled ileo-anal anastomosis without mucosectomy in restorative proctocolectomy. *Br J Surg* 1991;**78**:430–434

7   Luukkonen P, Jarvinen H. Stapled vs hand-sutured ileoanal anastomosis in restorative proctocolectomy: a prospective, randomized study. *Arch Surg* 1993; **128**:437–440

8   Wettergren A, Gyrtrup HJ, Grosmann E *et al.* Complications after J-pouch ileoanal anastomosis: stapled compared with handsewn anastomosis. *Eur J Surg* 1993;**159**:121–124

9   Lavery IC, Tuckson WB, Easley KA. Internal and sphincter function after total abdominal colectomy and stapled ileal pouch-anal anastomosis without mucosal proctocolectomy. *Dis Colon Rectum* 1989;**32**:950–953

10  Williams NS, Marzouk DEMM, Hallan RI, Waldron DJ. Function after ileal pouch and stapled pouch anal anastomosis for ulcerative colitis. *Br J Surg* 1989;**76**:1168–1171

11  Keighley MR. Abdominal mucosectomy reduces the incidence of soiling and sphincter damage after restorative proctocolectomy and J-pouch. *Dis Colon Rectum* 1998;**30**:386–390

12  Sugarman HJ, Newsome HH, DeCosta G, Zfass M. Stapled ileo-anal anastomosis for ulcerative colitis and familial polyposis without a temporary diverting ileostomy. *Ann Surg* 1991;**213**:606–619

13  Gullberg K, Lindquist K, Liljequist L. Pelvic pouch-anal anastomosis: pros and cons about omission of mucosectomy and loop ileostomy. A study of 60 patients. *Ann Chir* 1995;**49**:527–533

14  Johnston D, Holdsworth PJ, Nasmyth DG *et al.* Preservation of the entire anal canal in conservative proctocolectomy for ulcerative colitis – a pilot study comparing end-to-end ileo-anal anastomosis without mucosal resection, with mucosal proctectomy and endoanal anastomosis. *Br J Surg* 1987; **74**:940–944

15  Brant D, Cohen Z, McHugh S, McLeod RS, Stern H. Restorative proctocolectomy – clinical results and manometric findings. *Dis Colon Rectum* 1986; **29**:27–32

16  Ziv Y, Fazio VW, Sirimarco MT *et al.* Incidence, risk, factors and treatment of dysplasia in the anal transitional zone after ileal pouch-anal anastomosis. *Dis Colon Rectum* 1994;**37**:824–828

17  Heppell J, Weiland LH, Perrault J *et al.* Fate of the rectal mucosa after rectal mucosectomy and ileoanal anastomosis. *Dis Colon Rectum* 1983;**26**:768–771

18  Cohen Z, McLeod RS, Stephen W, Stern HS, O'Connor B, Reznick R. Continuing evolution of the pelvic pouch procedure. *Ann Surg* 1992;**21**:506–511

19  MacRae HM, McLeod RS, Cohen Z, O'Connor Bi, Ton ENC. Risk factors for pelvic pouch failure. *Dis Colon Rectum* 1997;**40**:257–262

20  Gemlo BT, Wong DW, Rothenberger DA, Goldberg SM. Ileal pouch-anal anastomosis: patterns of failure. *Arch Surg* 1992;**127**:784–787

21  Marcello PW, Roberts PL, Schoetz DL *et al.* Long-term results of the ileoanal pouch procedure. *Arch Surg* 1993;**128**:500–504

22  Matikainen M, Santavirta J, Hiltunen KM. Ileo-anal anastomosis without covering ileostomy. *Dis Colon Rectum* 1990;**33**:384–388

23  Galandiuk S, Wolff BG, Dozois RR, Beart RW Jr. Ileal pouch-anal anastomosis without ileostomy. *Dis Colon Rectum* 1991;**34**:870–873

24  Lohmuller JL, Pemberton JH, Dozois RR, Ilstrup D, van Heerden J. Pouchitis and extraintestinal manifestations of inflammatory bowel disease after ileal pouch-anal anastomosis. *Ann Surg* 1990;**221**:622–627

25  Madden MV, Farthing MJG, Nicholls RJ. Inflammation in ileal reservoirs: 'pouchitis.' *Gut* 1990;**31**:247–249

26  Pemberton JH, Kelly KA, Beart RW Jr *et al*. Ileal pouch anal anastomosis for chronic ulcerative colitis. Long term results. *Ann Surg* 1987;**206**:504–513

27  Stern H, Walfish S, Mullen B, McLeod RS, Cohen Z. Cancer in an ileo-anal reservoir – a new late complication. *Gut* 1990;**31**:473–475

28  Puthu D, Ragan N, Rao R, Rao L, Venugopal T. Carcinoma of the rectal pouch following restorative proctocolectomy report of a case. *Dis Colon Rectum* 1992;**35**:257–260

29  Hoehner JC, Metcalf AM. Development of invasive adenocarcinoma following colectomy with ileoanal anal anastomosis for familial polyposis coli. *Dis Colon Rectum* 1994;**37**:824–828

30  Cox CL, Butts DR, Roberts MP, Wessels RA, Bailey R. Development of invasive adenocarcinoma in a long standing Kock continent ileostomy. *Dis Colon Rectum* 1997;**40**:500–503

31  Rodriguez-Sanjuan JC, Polavieja MG, Naranjo A, Castillo J. Adenocarcinoma in an ileo-pouch for ulcerative colitis (letter). *Dis Colon Rectum* 1995;**38**:779–780

32  Smart PJ, Sastry S, Wells S. Primary mucinous adenocarcinoma developing in an ileostomy stoma. *Gut* 1998;**29**:1607–1612

33  Löfberg R, Liljeqvist L, Lindquist K, Veress B, Reinholt FP, Tribukait B. Dysplasia and DNA aneuploidy in a pelvic pouch – report of a case. *Dis Colon Rectum* 1991;**34**:280–284

34  Wu JS, Paul P, McGammon EA, Church JM. APC genotype, polyp number and surgical options in FAP. *Ann Surg* 1998;**1**:57–62

35  Rothenberger DA, Wong WD, Buls JG, Goldberg SM. The ileal pouch anal anastomosis. In: Dozors RR (ed) *Alternatives to Conventional Ileostomy*. Yearbook Med, Chicago

36  Richard CS, Cohen Z, Stern HS, McLeod RS. Outcome of the pelvic pouch procedure in patients with prior peri-anal diseases. *Dis Colon Rectum* 1997; **40**:647–652

37  McIntyre PB, Pemberton JH, Wolff BG *et al*. Indeterminate colitis – long-term outcome in patients after ileal pouch-anal anastomosis. *Dis Colon Rectum* 1995;**38**:51–54

38  Meagher AP, Farouk R, Dozors RR, Kelly KA, Pemberton JH. J ileal pouch-anal anastomosis for chronic uc: complications and long-term outcome in 1310 patients. *Br J Surg* 1998;**85**:800–803

39  Cohen Z, McLeod RS. Proctocolectomy and ileo-anal anastomosis with a J-shaped and s-shaped ileal pouch. *World J Surg* 1988;**12**:217–223

40  Oresland T, Fasth S, Nordgren S *et al*. The clinical and functional outcome after restorative proctocolectomy. A prospective study in 100 patients. *Int J Colorectal Dis* 1989;**4**:50–56

41  Lewis WG, Sagor PM, Holdsworth PJ *et al*. Restorative proctocolectomy with end-to-end pouch anal anastomosis in patients over the age of fifty. *Gut* 1993;**34**:948–952

42  Ojerskog D, Hallstrom T, Kock NG, Byrvold HE. Quality of life in patients before and after conversion to the continent ileostomy. *Int J Colorectal Dis* 1988;3:166–170

43  McLeod RS, Churchill DN, Lock AM, Vanderburgh S, Cohen Z. Quality of life of patients with ulcerative colitis preoperatively and postoperatively. *Gastroenterology* 1991;101:1307–1313

44  Jimmo B, Hymen NH. Is ileo-pouch anal anastomosis really the procedure of choice for patients with ulcerative colitis? *Dis Colon Rectum* 1998;41:41–45

45  Kohler LW, Pemberton JH, Zinmeister AR, Kelly KA. Quality of life after proctocolectomy: comparison of Brooke ileostomy, Kock pouch, and ileal pouch anal anastomosis. *Gastroenterology* 1991;101:679–681

# 9 What is the role of imaging in the management of colorectal cancer?

*Paul B Boulos, William R Lees and Alice Gillans*

## INTRODUCTION

Imaging techniques available for the evaluation of colorectal neoplasms include barium enema, endoscopy, computed tomography (CT), ultrasonography, magnetic resonance imaging (MRI), and immunoscintigraphy. In order to adopt a rational approach and appreciate the specific roles of the different methods, it is essential to recognize their benefits and limitations in the detection and staging of the primary cancer, in the assessment of systemic spread, and in the identification of disease recurrence after curative treatment.

## DIAGNOSIS OF THE PRIMARY CANCER AND DETECTION OF SYNCHRONOUS LESIONS

### Barium enema or colonoscopy?

The diagnostic maneuvers usually start with digital examination of the rectum and either rigid or flexible sigmoidoscopy. The advantage of rigid sigmoidoscopy is ease of performance and relatively low cost although in nearly half the patients it may not be possible to pass the instrument into the distal sigmoid because of patient discomfort or anatomic fixity. Alternatively, a flexible sigmoidoscope permits examination of a longer length of the distal large bowel with significant increase in the diagnostic yield, which is of particular importance because of the proximal shift in the distribution of colonic cancer. This feature is particularly relevant in the average risk patient with rectal bleeding as the sole symptom since complete visualization of the colon would be unnecessary unless a carcinoma or a polyp is evident in the segment examined. Synchronous polyps are found in

30–40% and approximately 5% of patients with colorectal cancer will have a synchronous cancer.

There is considerable debate as to the most appropriate method of complete colonic evaluation. In a review of the literature, Stevenson[1] concluded that the sensitivity of double-contrast barium enema (DCBE) in cancer detection was 65–99% compared with 70–95% in colonoscopy and found that for detecting polyps smaller than 1 cm, the best radiologic results were 85–90% compared with 90% for colonoscopy. For diminutive polyps, DCBE was only 40–60% accurate, whereas colonoscopy was 60–75% accurate. Thus, the performance of DCBE, although lower than colonoscopy, is sufficient to detect the majority of clinically important lesions.

An advantage of colonoscopy is that it allows identification and removal of any synchronous polyps before a planned resection for carcinoma. Certain features of adenomas predict subsequent risk of colorectal cancer; these traits include polyp size greater than 1 cm, multiplicity, villous or tubulovillous histology, and increasing levels of dysplasia.[2] Since the interval between adenoma and carcinoma appears to be approximately 5 years,[3] colonoscopy is particularly favored in younger patients. The benefit of colonoscopy in obtaining a tissue diagnosis is invaluable, since the radiologic appearances of a carcinoma are invariably diagnostic.

However, both methods have their limitations. Studies show that 5–10% of barium enemas are unsatisfactory, particularly in the very elderly and the seriously ill or in disabled patients who are usually less able to tolerate the procedure or retain the contrast material.[4] Barium enema will frequently fail to display the sigmoid colon in the presence of diverticular disease, when endoscopic examination is crucial to avoid missing neoplasia.[5] Similarly, the cecum is reached in 80–95% of procedures, depending on the experience of the endoscopist and the adequacy of the preparation.[6]

It is not clear which procedure patients consider more acceptable. Steine[7] found that patients who underwent both procedures rated pain significantly worse during colonoscopy compared with the barium enema. Williams *et al.*[8] found patients' preferences for the two procedures to be broadly similar, whereas Durdey *et al.*[9] and Van Ness *et al.*[10] found that more patients preferred colonoscopy. However, with the benefit of sedation, a well-prepared colon, and a skilled endoscopist, colonoscopy should be uneventful.

The most serious complication of barium enema is bowel perforation although the data are sparse, not current, and relate to single contrast. A retrospective, self-administered mail questionnaire estimated the perforation rate at 1 in 25 000 and cardiac complications at 1 in 46 000. However, the study has the weakness of self-reporting.[11]

Data from prospective studies of colonoscopy have indicated that approximately 1 in 1000 patients experience a perforation and 3 in 1000 major hemorrhage, and that 1–3 in 10 000 die as a result of the procedure. Complication rates may be higher if polypectomy is performed. Older patients do not seem to be at greater risk of complication than younger patients but they may tolerate the procedure less well.[12,13] About 5 in 1000 patients experience clinically significant respiratory depression.[14] Significant rhythm disturbance triggered by the procedure is rare.

Therefore, the choice between these two principal methods of diagnosis depends on the local expertise and the patient mix, and either is complementary to the other. If the tumor does not permit passage of a colonoscope proximally because of luminal narrowing, the proximal colon may be examined by a water-soluble contrast enema. However, if barium is forced through the stenotic segment, subsequent dehydration of the barium may precipitate colonic obstruction. Accordingly, water-soluble contrast is again much safer. Intraoperative palpation of the colon is inaccurate and colonoscopy at laparotomy can render mobilization difficult because of colonic distension. However, if carbon dioxide insufflation is employed, the problem of distention can be limited. When evaluation of the colon before operation is unsatisfactory, colonoscopy within 3 to 6 months after resection is advised.

## Does CT or ultrasonography have a role?

CT may incidentally identify a primary colorectal tumor but conventional cross-sectional imaging is unreliable for screening of intraluminal tumors and has been more useful in preoperative staging. However, CT has been recommended as the initial investigation in frail elderly patients based on a study of 36 such patients in whom the diagnosis was established in all six patients on CT and in five of six on barium enema.[15]

The introduction of helical CT has improved abdominal CT images, providing volumetric data, reduced motion artifact, better registration, and optimal vascular opacification. With intestinal cleansing, opacification and distension, imaging during the arterial phase of intravenous injection of contrast material, several thin section (5 mm) scans over the area of interest, and intravenous glucagon or Buscopan for bowel relaxation, imaging of colonic lesions is enhanced with a single breath hold scan of the abdomen. Several CT-based colon imaging techniques have now emerged which provide a promising novel approach to hollow organ evaluation.

Virtual colonoscopy involves interactive real-time helical CT data using high-performance computer software programs for image manipulation. By applying specific computer algorithms (perspective volume rendering algorithms) to helical datasets, an endoluminal 'flight-path' through any hollow organ can be traced, giving the observer a sense of motion through space in a manner similar to conventional colonoscopy without the need for sedation. Fenlon *et al.*,[16] using this technique, visualized the entire colon in 35 of 38 patients and correctly localized 38 cancers compared with 32 cancers localized by colonoscopy. Moreover, all polyps greater than 6 mm were also identified.

Helical or spiral CT pneumocolon, also known as CT colography, is another technique which involves dynamic intravenous contrast-enhanced thin-section helical CT of the air-insufflated colon with the aid of smooth muscle relaxants. CT data are displayed and interpreted using general purpose three-dimensional tools: multiplanar reformatting and three-dimensional volume rendering, when the two-dimensional base images require clarification. Harvey *et al.*,[17] using this technique, localized carcinoma in 37 patients and achieved an overall staging accuracy of 79% with a lymph node sensitivity of 56%. Hara and his colleagues[18] evaluated 30 endoscopically proven polyps in 10 patients and detected 100% of all polyps greater than 1 cm in diameter, 71% of polyps between 0.5 and 0.9 cm, and up to 28% of polyps less than 0.5 cm in size. This first study of CT for colon polyp detection shows promising results.

Regardless of the technology and terminology used, the clinical protocols for performing each of these CT techniques are essentially the same. All methods require thorough bowel cleansing, air insufflation of the colon, smooth muscle relaxation, helical CT acquisition, and some form of computer post-processing, with the only difference being the manner in which the helical CT data are manipulated and displayed. The benefits of this approach are that it involves a '60 second' examination, does not require sedation, and is noninvasive, which makes it particularly suitable for elderly and frail patients.

It may also provide a more complete examination of the colon than is possible with colonoscopy or barium enema when annular or constricting lesions are present. Finally, it can identify the extent of any liver and intra-abdominal involvement. However, there are inherent limitations related to misinterpretation, usually due to retained stool, poor distension, and difficulty in identifying flat lesions or subtle changes in mucosal color and texture, to be able to distinguish benign from malignant lesions. Although promising, the true potential of this approach requires a large-scale evaluation that takes into account the cost of software, hardware, reproducibility, learning curve time, and training.

Transabdominal ultrasound may pick up colonic cancer, especially in the right colon. Limberg[19] in Germany pioneered the use of hydrocolonic sonography, filling the prepared colon with water, and reported a detection rate of 97%, although the 91% rate of sensitivity of the technique in detecting polyps larger than 7 mm has been debated. A similar approach has been employed with MRI with promising results, but all hydrocolonic techniques are cumbersome.

## TUMOR STAGING

At present, accurate preoperative staging of the tumor does not influence the management of colonic cancer but is of particular relevance in rectal tumors as it determines the treatment plan. Careful evaluation defines those patients suitable for local excision or ablation therapy, those individuals with advanced but resectable cancers who will benefit from preoperative adjuvant radiotherapy, and those people with locally advanced cancers with extrarectal fixity and adjacent organ invasion where preoperative chemotherapy/radiotherapy may enhance resection. It is particularly helpful in identifying carcinomatous invasion in large villous adenomas, in order to decide on the extent of excision.

Clinical examination by digital assessment fails to determine early invasion into the rectal wall and the lymph node status but is more accurate in correctly assessing the stage of more advanced lesions where local excision would not be an option. The utilization of modern imaging in this respect has been widely explored and evaluated.

### Limitations of CT and MRI in tumor staging

CT and MRI have been employed in preoperative staging. A primary cancer appears as an area of circumferential bowel thickening and mass corresponding to the 'apple-core' appearance on a barium enema. Local invasion of tumor is suggested by soft tissue stranding and obliteration of the fascial planes or by extension of the mass into adjacent muscle, bone, or solid organ. However, these appearances are nonspecific, as inflammatory conditions such as diverticulitis or colitis may show similar features. Lymph node metastases are suspected by the finding of enlarged lymph nodes (>1 cm in diameter) which can be either reactive or malignant, whereas microscopic spread can occur within normal-sized lymph nodes and is not detectable by imaging. These limitations are responsible for the low reported sensitivity of CT: 53–77% in identification of local tumor extension and from 23 to 73% in detection of lymph node metastases.[20,21] The accuracy of CT appears to be stage dependent and is more accurate with advanced tumors, ranging from 17% for Dukes' B to 81% for infiltrating tumors.[22] MRI has similar limitations and sensitivity to those of CT, and has not proven to be superior to CT scanning in determining the penetration of tumor through the bowel wall or in assessing lymph node involvement, although extraluminal invasion is more clearly defined by MRI than by CT because of higher contrast between tumor and fat. As with CT, a standard body coil MRI does not demonstrate distinctly the layers of the bowel wall and is therefore of limited value in preoperative staging of rectal tumors.

## Staging of rectal tumors

The overall accuracy of MRI in the staging of rectal cancer using a body coil ranges from 59 to 95% and for nodal involvement from 39 to 95%.[23] An increased signal-to-noise ratio (SNR) is obtained by placing the coil closer to the region of interest; endoluminal and surface coils are used, such as the abdominal or pelvic phased-array multicoils. A dedicated endorectal coil allows increased resolution of the rectal wall and, similar to endosonography, can define the depth of invasion, which results in an improved and consistent accuracy rate of 75–90% for tumor staging.[24–26] Although MRI remains inferior to endoanal ultrasonography in tumor and nodal staging, it is the best modality for detecting tumor infiltration. A limitation of endoluminal imaging is a stricture that prevents optical imaging. A phased-array MRI is an alternative; it allows high-resolution visualization of the rectal tumor as well as distant metastases – without the need to introduce an intraluminal device – with an accuracy of 90%.[27,28]

Endorectal ultrasonography using rigid probes allows examination of the distal 12 cm of rectum with clear delineation of the different layers of the rectal wall. Accordingly, a tumor confined to the submucosa is $T_1$; once the muscularis propria is involved the tumor is $T_2$, and $T_3$ when the rectal wall is breached. With infiltration of an adjacent structure such as the prostate, the tumor is a $T_4$ stage. Reported correlation with histopathological tumor staging suggests an accuracy of 79–94%.[29] In a meta-analysis by Solomon and McLeod of 11 studies the sensitivities were 84%, 76%, 96%, and 76% for individual $T_{1-4}$ stages, respectively.[30] Overstaging is a particular problem with $T_2$ lesions, probably due to inflammatory changes around the tumor that are indistinguishable ultrasonographically from malignant infiltration. Understaging results from failure to detect microscopic infiltration because of the limited resolution. The accuracy of staging is also dependent on the level of the tumor, errors being more frequent in the lower rectum.[31,32] Staging is also less accurate following radiotherapy because of increased reflectivity in the tumor and the lymph nodes with loss of wall definition. Stenotic lesions are difficult to examine but may be staged with an 82% accuracy using a forward-viewing transducer.[33] Endorectal ultrasonography is less precise in lymph node staging. A meta-analysis has reported an outweighed kappa of 0.58 for detection of involved lymph nodes.[29] Complete tumor replacement will show typical ultrasonographic changes, but micrometastases will not alter the echogenicity or the configuration of the node. Invitro studies suggest a positive predictive value for nodal involvement of only 59%[34] and fewer than half the nodes in a resected specimen are visualized by endoanal ultrasonography.[35] Histologic verification when required can be obtained by ultrasound guided biopsy.[36]

Colonoscopic endoluminal ultrasonography has been used for staging tumors above the mid-rectum. This can be performed using an endoscope incorporating an ultrasonography transducer in the tip or by using an ultrasound probe introduced via the working channel of a conventional endoscope. In a recent report, accuracies of 92% and 65% were achieved in tumor and lymph node staging, respectively.[37]

Whereas endoanal ultrasonography is superior to CT and MRI in the T and N staging for rectal cancer, CT and MRI are better in staging advanced tumors and MRI is the best modality for detecting infiltration of other organs. Endoanal ultrasonography is particularly useful in selecting patients with $T_1$ or perhaps $T_2$ tumors for local excision and in distinguishing patients with villous adenomas for submucosal excision. The inaccuracy in lymph node detection is of no concern for $T_1$ but is for $T_2$ tumors, as lymph node involvement rises from less than 5% to 18%.[38]

## ASSESSMENT OF METASTASES

Pulmonary metastases are unusual and chest radiography is obtained as part of the preoperative assessment of the cardiorespiratory system. Common sites for early metastases from colorectal cancer include the liver and adrenal and retroperitoneal lymph nodes. Detection of metastatic disease inevitably alters the planned management.

### Choice and relevance of liver imaging

The liver is the commonest site of distant metastases. Surgery is the only therapy that offers cure, with a 5-year survival rate after resection of up to 40%. However, only 20–25% of patients with colorectal liver metastases are deemed suitable for hepatic resection.[39] Ablative therapies such as laser and radiofrequency have achieved a 5-year survival of 30% in patients with limited disease unsuitable for resection; for the remaining patients, treatment with regional or systemic chemotherapy, or any of the other new treatment modalities, can be expected to produce only modest extensions to survival time. The choice of therapy depends on the extent of liver involvement and, accordingly, precise imaging is required in a select group of patients considered suitable for additional treatment that can be scheduled at the time of resection of the primary tumor.

Ultrasonography of the liver is reasonably accurate for lesions larger than 2 cm; it is the least-expensive examination, and serves as a preliminary screening modality, particularly when adjuvant treatment is not anticipated, as in elderly or frail patients. Otherwise, should metastases be discovered in candidates elected for further treatment, better evaluation of the liver with MRI, CT angioportography (CTAP), or intraoperative ultrasonography is required, as the choice of treatment depends on the extent of the tumor bulk.

Intravenous iodinated contrast-enhanced CT scans are most sensitive because colorectal metastases, being supplied solely by the hepatic artery, are hypovascular and when portal venous opacification is at its peak, discrimination between the enhanced high-attenuation hepatic parenchyma and the lower-attenuation metastases is clearly evident. The reported sensitivity of CT for detection of hepatic metastases is in the range of 70 to 80%.[40] CT is least sensitive for detection of metastases less than 1 cm in diameter, but helical CT should reveal all lesions greater than 1 cm; the sensitivity of MRI is comparable to CT scans. Because of its greater cost, MRI is reserved for indeterminate lesions, since it provides improved characterization of lesions that can simulate metastases, such as focal fatty infiltration cysts or cavernous hemangiomas. Gadolinium-based intravenous contrast agents have been used in MRI examination to demonstrate the vascularity and enhancement pattern of such lesions and allow detection of small lesions. Liver-specific agents[41,42] are now available for MRI (superparamagnetic iron oxide particles and manganese difodipor) which allow detection of lesions of only a few millimeters in size but the specificity is poor. In addition, flow-sensitive MR images have been employed to define the vascular anatomy of the liver and helical CT angiography may prove to be of equal value in planning resectability of a lesion.

CTAP relies on the differential blood supply between the liver and hepatic tumors. Injection of iodinated contrast material into the portal venous system via a catheter positioned in the superior mesenteric artery results in a more selective portal phase scan than can be achieved with the peripheral vein injection. Hepatic metastases appear hypodense compared with the markedly enhanced hepatic parenchyma. Whereas CTAP has been regarded as most useful in detecting and localizing liver metastases for resection, intraoperative ultrasonography[43,44] and contrast enhanced MRI[41,42] are equally efficient. Helical CT performed with optimum technique[45] has a similar yield[46] and is probably the least invasive and most cost effective.

Intraoperative ultrasonography (IOUS) overcomes the problems inherent in percutaneous abdominal ultrasonography; by placing the transducer directly on the surface of the liver, a high frequency can be used, giving improved image quality, and intervening bowel loops can be avoided. A metastatic deposit as small as 5 mm in diameter can be diagnosed and appears as a hyperechoic lesion with a surrounding hypoechoic ring, described as a 'bull's-eye' appearance, although hypoechoic and isoechoic lesions have also been described. IOUS is the most sensitive modality in the detection of liver metastases (93–100%), compared with percutaneous ultrasonography (33–76%), CT (47–81%), angiography (38–52%), and surgical exploration (60–94%). Although the specificity is not different between the modalities, IOUS has the best overall accuracy.[47] The technique can be employed during laparotomy or laparoscopy.

Manual palpation and IOUS at laparotomy are complementary and, combined, provide the best measurement of liver metastases; they have been advocated for routine use. The inability to palpate the liver during laparoscopic colorectal cancer surgery has extended the role of IOUS, but laparoscopically guided IOUS remains unproven in comparison with open palpation and IOUS. Early experience has proven the feasibility and reliability of this approach.[48] Foley *et al.*[49] demonstrated a sensitivity of 94.4% and a specificity of 77.7% in an experimental pig model. In a human study, four of five liver metastases were detected and one was a single false negative: a specificity of 91%.[50] However, this technique may have limitations. There is difficulty in examining the entire surface area of the liver, especially over the liver dome, although this may be overcome with the use of a 30° laparoscope. Additionally, subcapsular lesions that are most frequently missed by IOUS and are detected by palpation are unlikely to be visible at laparoscopic ultrasonography.[50,51]

## Prediction of risk of developing liver metastases

It has been argued that IOUS does not confidently identify those patients who may develop hepatic metastases in the long term (patients with false-negative scans) and, therefore, does not provide a survival benefit. In follow-up data presented by Machi *et al.*,[52] three (7%) of 189 patients had developed hepatic metastases 18 months after primary resection that had not been detected at the time of the initial surgery by any modality including IOUS. Leen *et al.*[53] found that at 2-year follow up, 22 (23.6%) of 93 patients that had been examined by IOUS developed liver metastases. Paul *et al.*[54] reported a 16% incidence of liver metastases at 2 years after negative IOUS examination on 85 patients. Evidence is accumulating from Doppler ultrasound and dynamic CT that occult liver metastases alter the ratio of hepatic arterial and portal venous blood supply to the liver.[55,56] The Doppler perfusion index (i.e. the ratio of hepatic arterial to total liver blood flow) identifies those patients with a high risk of subsequent development of metastases and, therefore, who may benefit from adjuvant chemotherapy.[53] However, the technique is difficult, fails to yield specific sites of recurrence, and promising early results have proven difficult to reproduce.

## IMAGING IN FOLLOW UP AND DETECTION OF DISEASE RECURRENCE

The intensity of follow up takes into account prognostic indicators that are the pathologic features of the tumor and clinical factors associated with patient survival and recurrence, which include age, gender, and presence of obstruction or perforation. It is estimated that 39–50% of colorectal cancers will recur after curative resection[21] and 80% of recurrences present within 2 years of the initial resection.[19] Hepatic metastases account for almost 50% of recurrence, local recurrence at the area of bowel resection for about 33%, and peritoneal seedlings for 22%.[21] Early treatment may improve patient survival. Imaging strategies are employed accordingly and are aimed at demonstrating local recurrence and distant metastases to determine the most appropriate management approach.

## Early detection of a second primary

When evaluation of the colon for synchronous lesions before operation is unsatisfactory, it is usually done within 3 to 6 months after resection, then every 5 years or more frequently in patients who had synchronous cancer or with hereditary nonpolyposis colorectal cancer (HNPCC) in order to detect early metachronous tumors. The therapeutic benefit of colonoscopy when polyps are detected makes it the first choice. However, when the colon is clear, barium enema or virtual colonoscopy or any of the related CT techniques is a reliable noninvasive alternative, reserving colonoscopy for therapeutic intervention.

## Anastomotic recurrence

A recurrence at an anastomosis rarely originates from tumor growth at the suture line and is usually due to tumor infiltration arising from recurrent disease in the lymphovascular tissues in the vicinity of an anastomosis. Therefore, luminal distortion from extrinsic tumor growth may be more prominent than mucosal infiltration and an anastomotic recurrence may herald the presence of peritoneal or pelvic recurrence. These are relevant considerations for designing the appropriate imaging of the area of interest.

Anastomotic recurrence is infrequent after ileocolic or colocolic anastomosis and when it manifests clinically it is morphologically identifiable by either a barium enema or colonoscopy. The anastomotic area is narrowed, asymmetric, and irregular, and extrinsic compression may be evident. CT outlines the extent of extraluminal disease, which appears as a discrete mass or local infiltration into neighboring structures of fascial planes. Histologic confirmation is obtained directly from the mucosa, if clearly involved; otherwise, confirmation is by an ultrasound- or CT-guided needle biopsy of the tumor mass.

Anastomotic recurrence is more common after a colorectal or coloanal anastomosis; it is extrarectal and is a component of a pelvic recurrence. Anastomotic recurrence is detectable by endoanal ultrasonography before it is discernible by digital palpation or sigmoidoscopy, when by then it is irresectable to justify regular follow-up examination after sphincter-preserving resection for rectal cancer.[57]

## Peritoneal and pelvic recurrence

CT is the most useful imaging study for the overall postoperative screening of the abdomen and pelvis and will detect extraluminal recurrence and lymphadenopathy or peritoneal seeding. However, MRI is less sensitive for evaluation of extraluminal tumor recurrence and peritoneal implants.

Local recurrence following curative resection for rectal cancer occurs in 10–30%[58] of patients. The early detection of local pelvic recurrence has been emphasized because of favorable survival rates that may be achieved by extended radical operations such as pelvic exenteration.[59,60] CT is of particular importance in the postoperative follow up of patients who have had abdominoperineal resection for rectal carcinoma and is more sensitive in the diagnosis of local recurrence after abdominoperineal resection than after restorative resection. Clinical symptoms of recurrence are nonspecific and generally present only when the disease is advanced after direct invasion of adjacent structures. Rectal excision precludes digital or endoscopic examination, although transvaginal digital and ultrasonographic evaluation may be useful. Local recurrence most often manifests as a presacral mass that spreads locally to involve the pelvic organs and bones. The appearance on CT is of an irregular heterogeneous soft tissue density presacral mass with ill-defined margins that may be indistinguishable from postoperative changes such as fibrosis hematoma or abscess. Postoperative radiotherapy to the pelvis results in fibrous tissue reaction which shows on CT as linear streaky soft tissue density in the presacral and pelvic fat, very similar to the CT appearance of tumor recurrence. The diagnostic accuracy is improved with a baseline study obtained early in the postoperative period at 3 months[1,18] after abdominoperineal resection for comparison with subsequent follow-up scans obtained every 6 months for 2 years, then annually if the patient remains disease-free. CT-guided percutaneous needle biopsy will aid in evaluating the diagnosis; however, such an approach may be tempered by the significant cost of CT scanning.

MRI is more accurate in the diagnosis of recurrence in up to 80% of patients.[61] On MRI, most malignant tumors have intermediate-to-high signal intensity, whereas fibrous tissue has low signal intensity. The sensitivity of MRI in detection of local recurrence is reportedly from 80 to 91% with specificity as high as 100% compared with 82% sensitivity and 50% specificity for CT.[61] However, its discriminatory ability may be disturbed by high signal intensity produced by abscesses, fluid collection, or inflammatory changes, or when the tumor is interspersed within inflammatory or fibrous tissue that interfere with the intensity of the signal. Because of these imaging limitations, CT-guided biopsy may still be required.

Although CT and MRI have both been effective in detecting pelvic recurrence, the recurrence is not recognized until it is large. Although periodic examination using CT and MRI is indicative of tumor recurrence, these tests do not provide sufficiently early detection and the patient may lose the opportunity to undergo curative resection. In this respect, positron emission tomography (PET) and immuno-scintigraphy have more to offer. Conversely, they are less widely available and possibly more expensive.

## Hepatic metastases

Liver imaging is either routinely performed as part of the follow-up strategy or when the carcinoembryonic antigen (CEA) level shows a rise. The choice of the imaging method will largely depend on the suitability of the patient for active treatment. Ultrasonography is readily available and inexpensive but has a sensitivity of less than 60% for individual colorectal metastases; often, even large metastases are missed. It is, therefore, inadequate if treatment – considered as the benefit of any form of therapy, either surgical or local palliative – is dependent on a precise measure of the extent of liver involvement. However, recently, gray-scale sonography with a high-end ultrasound system has been reported to have a similar potential to CT for screening liver metastases.[62] Helical CT with its high sensitivity[45,46] should detect all liver secondaries more than 1 cm in size and will determine the suitability for resection by demonstrating the number and distribution of secondaries and absence of extrahepatic recurrence. In an early study[63] the sensitivities of CTAP, delayed CT, lipid-enhanced CT, and MRI were comparable at around 85% for all lesions, and

95–97% for lesions over 2 cm in diameter, but MRI was superior, as it had the lowest false-positive rate. In clinical practise, helical CT is adequate, MRI is helpful for lesion characterization or preoperative assessment, and CTAP is infrequently used, although several studies have emphasized its superiority in detection of lesions 1 cm or less in diameter and the benefit it provides when assessing operability.[64–66]

IOUS is particularly useful in the localization and assessment of resectability of liver lesions. In several reports, IOUS detected lesions not found by preoperative investigation or liver palpation in a significant number of patients (9–29%) and influenced surgical decision-making in between 32 and 51% of planned liver resections.[67–72] Ultrasonography is particularly useful in finding lesions rendered impalpable by cirrhotic nodularity.[67] It accurately delineates the proximity to or invasion of the hepatic vasculature, which allows avoiding resection when invasion is proven or modification of the resection when the vessels are clear. In some centers, ultrasonography is routinely employed.

Chest CT is often used to exclude lung metastases in patients with potentially resectable liver metastases. However, it has been shown that the majority of lesions appearing on the chest CT scans of patients with negative chest radiographs are malignant in only 5% of cases.[73]

Radioimmunoscintigraphy and PET, as described later, may have an exclusive role in a few patients in order to rule out extrahepatic disease when resectional heptic surgery is being considered, as they have the capacity of identifying early recurrence with high accuracy.

### Imaging in the treatment of liver metastases

Hepatic artery chemoembolization[74] was developed as a treatment for unresectable localized metastases and has been utilized to cause sufficient tumor shrinkage to allow resection and to decrease perioperative tumor dissemination, but this has not been substantiated. Portal vein embolization by percutaneous ultrasonography-guided puncture of a portal vein radicle (through tumor-free liver) has been advocated in order to decrease the likelihood of liver insufficiency occurring after extensive liver resection by inducing hypertrophy in the future remnant liver.[75] Brachytherapy with yttrium-90 microspheres or iodine-125 seeds has been used with favorable responses in patients with irresectable colorectal metastases.[76] As an alternative to direct surgical implantation, radioactive material has been applied in a relatively selective fashion by combining the radioisotope with

Lipoidal with delivery by radiologic embolization.[77] Hepatic arteriography is routinely employed to define any anatomic aberration in the vasculature in order to allow safe catheterization of the hepatic artery for regional infusion chemotherapy in patients with irresectable liver metastases. Any of the imaging modalities – ultrasonography, CT, and MRI, depending on the individual case – is suitable to provide percutaneous access for ablation of irresectable liver lesions, with ethanol, laser interstitial hyperthermia, cryotherapy, or radiofrequency.

## Other visceral metastases

In the absence of liver metastases, pulmonary, cerebral, or bony metastases are rare and routine screening is not employed unless clinically indicated.

# IMPROVING THE DIAGNOSTIC ACCURACY OF RECURRENCE

The limitations of CT and MRI with respect to detectable tumor size and specificity, and the difficulty in distinguishing a post-surgical or post-radiotherapy fibrosis, an inflammatory mass, or a recurrence, may be resolved with diagnostic modalities that depend on the biological characteristics of malignant cells. In this respect, radioimmunoscintigraphy (RIS) and PET fulfil this requirement.

## Radioimmunoscintigraphy

The clinical application of radiolabeled antibodies has been evaluated in several studies. A variety of antibodies (CEA, B72.3, and PR1A3), antigen targets, radiolabels (iodine-123, indium-111, technetium-99mc), and imaging protocols have been used. The B72.3 antibody labeled with indium-111 is available commercially (Oncoscint). Its main drawback is that up to 20% of colorectal cancers do not express the TAG-72 antigen so at best sensitivity is only 80%, whereas PR1A3 labeled with indium-111 or technetium-99mc reacts with 97% of colorectal cancers as does the anti-CEA antibody.[78–80]

RIS using [111]In-labeled CYT103, an immunoconjugate of monoclonal antibody B72.3, was evaluated in 155 patients with primary or recurrent colorectal cancers at 25 centers in the United States.[81] RIS and CT showed similar sensitivity (69% vs 68%) and specificity (77%). However, RIS had greater sensitivity in detection of pelvic tumors (74% vs 57%) and extrahepatic abdominal tumors (66% vs 34%). CT detected a greater proportion of liver metastases (84% vs 41%). In another coordinated research program[82] the overall accuracy of RIS using technetium-99mc labeled BW 431/26, a monoclonal antibody against CEA in the diagnosis of recurrence, was 87%. Its sensitivity in detection of locoregional or abdominal recurrence and liver metastases was 97% and 89%, respectively. RIS was more accurate than CT in the detection of pelvic recurrence and liver metastases. Intraoperative use of a gamma probe in tracing recurrence has further allowed the detection of 'micrometastatic deposits'.[83] Other studies have corroborated the diagnostic benefit of RIS in the management of recurrent disease.[84,85]

## Positron emission tomography

PET scanning with fluorine deoxyglucose (FDG), a glucose substitute taken up by cancer cells, detects increased FDG uptake in recurrent cancer (soft tissue mass seen on CT). In a comparison of FDG-PET with CT, MRI, and RIS, despite the small numbers, PET demonstrated greater sensitivity and specificity than the other methods.[86–88] Schiepers *et al.*[89] investigated 76 patients with suspected recurrent local or distant disease by PET, CT pelvis, CT liver, ultrasonography, and chest radiology. The accuracy of PET for local disease was superior to CT pelvis (95% vs 65%) for liver metastases and compared favorably with CT and ultrasonography (98% vs 93%). Unexpected extrahepatic metastases were detected by PET in 14 sites in 10 patients. Delbeke *et al.*[90] identified 166 suspicious lesions in 52 patients with suspected recurrence: of 127 intrahepatic lesions, 104 were malignant; and of the 39 extrahepatic lesions, 34 were malignant. FDG-PET was more accurate (92%) than CT and CTAP (78% and 80%) in detecting liver metastases and more accurate than CT for extrahepatic metastases (92% and 71%). FDG-PET detected unsuspected metastases in 17 patients and altered surgical management in 28% of patients. Tukeuchi *et al.*[91] have further shown that it is possible to distinguish recurrent lesions from non-malignant masses with a high degree of accuracy by optimizing the tracer uptake measurement.

Although several reports have demonstrated the capability of RIS and PET in detecting primary colorectal cancer and liver metastases, the cost effectiveness of current conventional modalities make their contribution in this respect superfluous. The main impact of RIS and PET is their ability to identify early peritoneal or pelvic recurrence not within the resolution of CT and MRI. They are particularly of value in patients with rising CEA levels on clinical follow up in whom other imaging methods have failed. However, they bear two distinct limitations. First, an inflammatory mass will show monoclonal antibody uptake although this will fade with time, whereas it will progress with recurrent tumor. Similarly, since PET reflects the metabolic activity of tissues, it is difficult to differentiate malignant tissue from active inflammation because glucose metabolism in the leukocytes is activated. Secondly, the configuration of the tumor and involvement of other structures cannot be defined unless CT or MRI are combined to provide a precise anatomic image.

## SUMMARY

Colonoscopy and DCBE are the conventional investigations for the diagnosis of colorectal cancer and synchronous neoplasms. Helical CT pneumocolon or colography is a promising new technique that allows complete examination of the colon combined with clinical staging. Although CT and MRI have a low sensitivity for outlining local tumor extension and lymph node involvement, CT is superior to MRI in defining extrahepatic metastases. Endoluminal ultrasonography and, to a lesser extent endoluminal MRI, are the best methods for measuring the depth of invasion within the rectal wall. The diagnostic efficacy of helical CT, MRI, CTAP, and IOUS in the detection of hepatic metastasis provides a choice for the individual case and proposed extent of management. CTAP is recommended before resection of solitary metastases and IOUS delineates the hepatic vasculature and allows adequate oncological clearance (Tables 9.1 and 9.2).

A standard follow-up protocol includes CEA and ultrasonography of the liver, although CT is preferable when additional treatment is planned. A baseline CT scan of the pelvis after abdominoperineal excision of the rectum and every 6 months for 2 years, and then annually, and, similarly, transrectal ultrasonography after sphincter-preserving resection improves the diagnostic accuracy of early recurrence. PET scan and immunoscintigraphy are more sensitive than CT and MRI in distinguishing peritoneal or pelvic recurrence from postoperative changes; however, their cost and relative lack of global penetration limits their utility.

**Table 9.1** Summary of investigational strategy

| | |
|---|---|
| Primary diagnosis | Colonoscopy or DCBE (CT) colography for incomplete studies, frail and elderly |
| **Staging** | |
| *Local* | Rectal tumors only |
| | Endoluminal US/MRI |
| | Helical CT |
| *Liver metastases* | MRI with a liver-specific contrast agent |
| | Intraoperative US |
| **Recurrence** | |
| *Liver* | Helical CT |
| *Pelvic* | PET |
| | Helical CT |
| | MRI |

CT, computed tomography; DCBE, double-contrast barium enema; MRI, magnetic resonance imaging; PET, positron emission tomography; US, ultrasonography.

**Table 9.2** Advantages and disadvantages of different imaging modalities

| Modality | Advantages | Disadvantages |
|---|---|---|
| Abdominal US | Inexpensive | Poor sensitivity |
| | Widely available | Dependent on patient body habitus |
| Endoanal US | Useful for $T_1/T_2$ staging | Local information only |
| Helical CT | Less expensive than MRI | No demonstration of |
| | Provides a more comprehensive | bowel wall layers, even with |
| | assessment of the abdomen | the latest colographic techniques |
| | and pelvis | Inability to distinguish pelvic fibrosis |
| | Reasonable detection rates | from recurrence |
| CTAP | Very high sensitivity | Invasive |
| | | Low specificity – has largely been |
| | | abandoned in favor of helical |
| | | CT or MRI |
| MRI | Multiplanar | Not widely available |
| | Superior soft tissue contrast | Expensive |

**Table 9.2** *(continued)*

| Modality | Advantages | Disadvantages |
| --- | --- | --- |
| | Liver-specific contrast agent, enhanced MRI, best noninvasive method for detection of liver metastases | Time consuming, therefore used to answer specific questions |
| | Can differentiate fibrosis from recurrence in the pelvis | |
| PET | Better detection of pelvic recurrence than CT or MRI | Very expensive |
| | | Restricted availability |
| | | Nonspecific in the presence of inflammation |

CT, computed tomography; CTAP, computed tomography angioportography; MRI, magnetic resonance imaging; PET, positron emission tomography; US, ultrasonography.

# REFERENCES

1   Stevenson GW. Medical imaging in the prevention, diagnosis and management of colon cancer. In: Herlinger H, Megibow A J (eds) *Advances in Gastrointestinal Radiology*. Mosby Year Book, St Louis, 1991, pp 1–20

2   Atkin WS, Morson BG, Cuzick J. Long term risk of colorectal cancer after excision of rectosigmoid adenomas. *N Engl J Med* 1992;326:658–662

3   Winawer SJ, Zauber AG, Diaz B. The National Polyp Study; temporal sequence of evolving colorectal cancer from the normal colon. *Gastrointest Endosc* 1987;33: A167

4   Bloomfield JA. Reliability of barium enema in detecting colonic neoplasia. *Med J Aust* 1981;1:631–633

5   Boulos PB, Karamanolis DG, Salmon PR, Clark CG. Is colonoscopy necessary in diverticular disease? *Lancet* 1984;1:95–96

6   Anderson ML, Neigh RI, McCoy GA *et al*. Accuracy of assessment of the extent of examination by experienced colonoscopists. *Gastrointest Endosc* 1992;38: 560–563

7   Steine S. Which hurts the most? A comparison of pain rating during double-contrast barium enema examination and colonoscopy. *Radiology* 1994;191:99–101

8   Williams CB, Macrae FA, Bartram CA. A prospective study of diagnostic methods in adenoma follow-up. *Endoscopy* 1982;14:74–78

9   Durdey P, Weston PMT, Williams NS. Colonosopy or barium enema as initial investigation of colonic disease. *Lancet* 1987;2:549–551

10  Van Ness MM, Chobanian SJ, Winters C Jr, Diehl AM, Esposito RL, Cattau EL Jr. A study of patient acceptance of double-contrast barium enema and colonoscopy.

79  Lind P, Lechner P, Arian-Schad K *et al.* Anti-carcinoembryonic antigen immunoscintigraphy (technetium-99[m] monoclonal antibody BW431/26) and serum CEA levels in patients with suspected primary and recurrent colorectal carcinoma. *J Nucl Med* 1991;**32**:1319–1325

80  Granowska M, Mather SJ, Britton KE. Diagnostic evaluation of [111]In and 99[m]Tc radiolabelled monoclonal antibodies in ovarian and colorectal cancer: correlations with surgery. *Nucl Med Biol* 1991;**18**:413–424

81  Collier BD, Abdel-Nabi H, Doerr RJ *et al.* Immunoscintigraphy performed with In-111 labelled CYT-103 in the management of colorectal cancer: comparison with CT. *Radiology* 1992;**185**:179–186

82  Poshyachinda M, Chaiwatanarat T, Saesow N, Thitathan S, Voravud N. Value of radioimmunoscintigraphy with technetium-99m labelled anti-CEA monoclonal antibody (BW431\26) in the detection of colorectal cancer. *Eur J Nucl Med* 1996;**23**:624–630

83  Cote RJ, Houchens DP, Hitchcock CL *et al.* Intra-operative detection of occult colon cancer mucometastasis using [125]I-radiolabelled monoclonal antibody CC49. *Cancer* 1996;**77**:613–620

84  Divgi CR, McDermott K, Griffin TW *et al.* Lesion by lesion comparison of computerized tomography and indium-111 labelled monoclonal antibody C110 radioimmunoscintigraphy in colorectal carcinoma: a multicentre trial. *J Nucl Med* 1993;**34**:1656–1661

85  Lunniss PJ, Skinner S, Britton KE, Granowska M, Morris G, Northover JMA. Effect of radioimmunoscintigraphy in the management of recurrent colorectal cancer. *Br J Surg* 1999;**85**:244–249

86  Gupta N, Boman B, Frank A *et al.* PET FDG imaging for follow-up evaluation of treated colorectal cancer. *Radiology* 1991;**181**(suppl):199(abstract)

87  Ito K, Kato T, Tadokoro M *et al.* Recurrent colorectal cancer and scar: differentiation with PET and MR imaging. *Radiology* 1992;**182**:549–552

88  Schlag P, Lehner B, Strauss LG, Georgi P, Herfarth C. Scar or recurrent rectal cancer: positron emission tomography is more helpful for diagnosis than immunoscintigraphy. *Arch Surg* 1989;**124**:197–200

89  Schiepers C, Pennickx F, DeVadder N *et al.* Contribution of PET in the diagnosis of recurrent colorectal cancer: comparison with conventional imaging. *Eur J Surg Oncol* 1995;**21**:517–522

90  Delbeke D, Vitola JV, Sandler MP *et al.* Staging recurrent metastatic colorectal carcinoma with PET. *J Nucl Med* 1997;**38**:1196–1201

91  Takeuchi O, Saito N, Koda K, Sarashina H, Nakajima N. Clinical assessment of positron emission tomography for the diagnosis of local recurrence in colorectal cancer. *Br J Surg* 1999;**86**:932–937

# 10 How can the surgeon improve the outcome in rectal cancer?

*Robert J C Steele*

## INTRODUCTION

The main aim of rectal cancer surgery is to remove the primary tumor in such a way as to minimize the risk of locoregional recurrence. The role of adjuvant radiotherapy in this respect is currently much debated; a number of randomized trials have demonstrated the effectiveness of preoperative[1,2] and postoperative[3] radiotherapy, but the local recurrence rates in the control arms of all of these studies were considerably higher than those achieved by surgery alone in several single institution series.[4–8] The reasons for this observation can be debated, but in this chapter, the pros and cons of adjuvant radiotherapy is not being examined. Rather, the emphasis is on the specific role of surgery.

The surgeon's second important goal is to ensure that the quality of life experienced after rectal cancer surgery is acceptable. In general, this is taken to mean avoiding a permanent stoma, and this can be done either by a reconstructive procedure after rectal excision, anterior resection, or by means of local excision of the tumor. However, it must be appreciated that, in a number of patients, the best quality of life is provided by a stoma, and appropriate patient selection for either of these procedures is essential.

Surgery for rectal cancer is technically demanding, and as surgical excision is still the most important component of curative treatment, it is likely that the surgeon will be highly influential in determining outcome in this disease. In considering how the surgeon can improve the outcome for a patient with rectal cancer it is important first to look at technique and how this relates to results, and secondly to examine how the choice of operation relates to outcome, both in terms of locoregional recurrence and quality of life. Finally, we analyze the evidence for surgeon-related variation and the effect of volume and specialization.

floor. Many surgeons use the 'triple staple' method, which involves placing a row of staples across the distal rectum below the tumor, washing out the rectal stump below this with a cytocidal agent introduced per anum and then placing a further row of staples distal to the first row. The rectum is divided immediately above the second row of staples by using a long-handled knife to divide immediately flush with the cephalad side of the linear stapler after it is fired, but before it is released. The very short rectal stump is then ready for anastomosis using a circular end-to-end stapler, and the likelihood of tumor cells being incorporated into the staple line is minimized by the washout. After resection, inspection of the specimen should reveal a

**Fig 10.5** Posterior view of specimen after anterior resection with total mesorectal excision. Note the intact mesorectum and distal staple line.

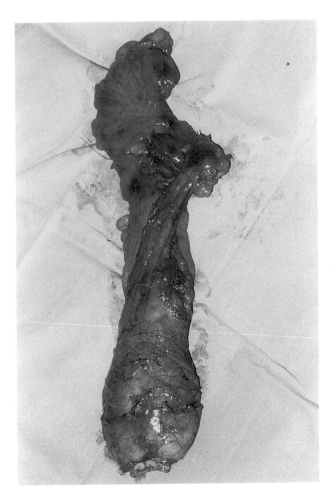

bulky mesorectum, with an intact fascial covering and no underlying rectal muscle should be seen (Fig. 10.5).

It must be emphasized that abdominoperineal excision of rectum (APER) for a very low tumor is not an alternative to TME. Rather, an APER must incorporate all the features of TME as described above with the exception of division of the distal rectum. Conversely, when a tumor is situated in the upper third of the rectum, it is generally accepted that TME is unnecessary and that transection of the mesorectum 5 cm below the lower limit of the tumor is safe. However, it must be stressed that dissection in the correct plane just outside the mesorectum remains an essential component of the operation.

Evidence that these principles are effective in minimizing local recurrence emerges from single surgeon series. The foremost proponent of TME is Heald, and in 1993 an independent assessor reviewed all the prospectively collected data from his patients undergoing this procedure.[4] No patient had adjuvant radiotherapy or chemotherapy. A subgroup of patient with Dukes' stage B and C undergoing curative resections was analyzed, and the local recurrence rate at 5 years was 5% with an overall recurrence rate of 22%. Heald's results are not unique, and other groups using identical or similar surgical techniques for rectal cancer have obtained comparable results. In Sweden, the specialist colorectal group for the county of Oster-gotland obtained an overall local recurrence rate of 6%.[7] Enker et al.[5] from New York have reported a local recurrence rate of 7.3%, Marks et al.[6] from England a rate of 8%, and Aitken[8] from Edinburgh a rate of 2% at 2 years. Wexner and associates have noted similar results by assiduous routine utilization of the TME dissection (unpublished data).

TME is not without its problems, however, and there is at least one report of a high local recurrence rate – almost 20% after 45 potentially curative procedures.[14] This highlights the difficulty in categorizing surgical expertise merely by operative nomenclature; one surgeon's TME may be very different from that of another.

A more consistent disadvantage of TME, and therefore more serious, is the associated anastomotic dehiscence rate. Heald et al. reported a 17.4% leak rate,[15] Aitken 14%,[8] Hainsworth et al. 19%,[14] and the Norwegian group noted an increase from 8% to 16% after the introduction of TME.[16] The reasons for this are not clear, but Heald noted that the use of a defunctioning stoma lessened the risk of a major leak, and that the use of sigmoid rather than descending colon for the anastomosis was associated with a higher dehiscence rate.[15] Despite some better results,[5] the anastomotic leak rate commonly experienced after TME is higher than the 8% rate after anterior resection reported by the unselected audit of all colorectal cancer surgery in the Wales and Trent region in 1992–1993,[17] and considerably higher than the best in the literature.[18] This would seem to indicate that, with present techniques, TME is generally associated with a higher anastomotic leak rate than is conventional anterior resection, and that defunctioning is a wise precaution for most surgeons at least.

Even more radical surgery than TME, involving lateral lymph node dissection beyond the limits of the mesorectum, is practiced, especially in Japan.[19] The main problem with this approach is nerve damage and consequent bladder and sexual dysfunction. In men, sacrifice of the superior hypogastric plexus leads to failure of ejaculation and preservation of the inferior hypogastric plexus is necessary to avoid impotence.[20] For this reason, radical pelvic lymphadenectomy has been dismissed for routine use in the West, but recent technical modifications have made it possible to combine nerve preservation with radical pelvic node dissection.[20] As yet, however, no clear advantage over mesorectal excision has been demonstrated.

## IMPROVING THE FUNCTIONAL OUTCOME AFTER RECTAL CANCER SURGERY

Although avoiding a permanent stoma is often taken as a *sine qua non* for a good outcome after rectal cancer surgery, functional success must be considered separately. Frequency of bowel action, diarrhea, urgency, fecal leakage, incontinence, and even constipation, can be present in varying degrees after anterior resection, and a low colorectal or coloanal anastomosis is associated with worse functional results than a high anterior resection.[21] The erratic bowel function due to a rectal tumor may not improve after low anterior resection,[22] which suggests that some patients may be better served by a permanent stoma. Unfortunately, there are no reliable means whereby function after low anterior resection can be predicted; anorectal physiology studies have been largely restricted to postoperative studies, and show that poor function is associated with low anal sphincter pressures and abnormal rectoanal inhibitory reflexes that do not improve with time.[21] It makes sense, however, to avoid attempting a low anterior resection on a patient with poor sphincter function.

However, given that an individual is likely to achieve a better quality of life with a reconstructive procedure after rectal excision, an abdominoperineal excision of the rectum should be avoided if at all possible. The 'old rule' of ensuring that 5 cm of distal clearance is achieved has now been rendered redundant; careful histologic studies have shown that distal intramural spread is rare, and if it occurs for more that 1 cm the patient will almost certainly have distant metastases.[23] In addition, Heald's work has shown that, as long as TME is performed, a 'close shave' anterior resection where a clamp or stapler is placed just distal to the tumor and the rectal stump washed out with a cytocidal agent before applying the definitive staple line across the anorectal junction will achieve excellent local control.[24] This must not be confused with mesorectal *transection* where distal clearance of 5 cm is essential, as performed for tumors in the upper third of the rectum.

When an anterior resection is to be performed there are certain steps the surgeon can take to maximize the chances of acceptable function. As a high anastomosis is associated with better results, one important principle is to avoid coloanal anastomosis if this is not necessary. If TME is not required to achieve local control (i.e. if the mesorectum can be safely transected at least 5 cm distal to the tumor), then as much of a rectal stump as possible should be preserved. If, however, a TME is necessary then the stapled coloanal anastomosis can be performed using a short, 5 cm, 'J' pouch created out of the distal descending or sigmoid colon. This measure may improve function by increasing the threshold and maximum tolerable volumes of the neorectum.[25,26] There have been at least two randomized trials comparing pouches with straight coloanal anastomoses that have demonstrated a better functional outcome with the use of a pouch.[27,28] It must be emphasized, however, that pouches can be associated with difficulty in evacuation, especially if the pouch is large or if it has been anastomosed to an appreciable rectal remnant.[29,30]

The other approach to improving functional outcome is to undertake a local excision of the tumor, usually by the transanal route. Few surgeons would advocate this procedure in cases of early ($T_1$) lesions where an anterior resection can be safely performed with a reasonable expectation of acceptable function, but in selected cases, especially where an abdominoperineal resection is the only alternative, local excision may be appropriate. Tumors suitable for local excision must be accessible, small ($\leqslant 3$ cm), and confined to the rectal wall. They should not show anaplastic histology. Transanal endoscopic surgery has allowed access to the upper rectum and increases the scope for local excision.

The main problem with this approach is the high risk of locoregional recurrence when compared with the results that can be obtained with radical surgery.[31] Even with a $T_1$ tumor, the overall risk of regional lymph node involvement by tumor may be as much as 10%,[32] and with $T_2$ and $T_3$ tumors these figures are around 20% and 50%, respectively.[33] However, $T_1$ tumors can be subclassified as high- or low-risk on the basis of histologic differentiation and lymphovascular invasion,[34] and most surgeons would accept local excision of a low-risk $T_1$ lesion as adequate therapy.

There has been one randomized trial of local excision versus radical surgery for rectal cancers preoperatively diagnosed as $T_1$ tumors by transrectal ultrasound.[35] In this study, the patients undergoing local excision fared significantly better in terms of immediate postoperative outcome (i.e. blood loss, analgesia requirement, length of hospitalization), and there was no significant difference in locoregional recurrence at 40 months. However, there was one locoregional recurrence in the locally treated group and none in the radically operated group, and as there were only 26 patients in each arm of the trial, the study had insufficient power to prove equivalence between the two techniques in terms of this complication.

Despite the lack of convincing randomized evidence, there is an increasing tendency to treat $T_{1-2}$ tumors by local excision, usually with pre- or postoperative radiotherapy often combined with chemotherapy.[35-38] A relatively high locoregional recurrence rate must be accepted if this approach is to be adopted, but with careful follow up using transrectal ultrasound and prompt salvage surgery, the centers which publish their results seem to achieve acceptable disease-free survival. Clearly, if this method is to be practiced, it must be undertaken with extreme care and fully informed consent from the patient. Adequately powered randomized trials will be difficult to perform in this area, but if local excision is to enter the mainstream of surgical practice as a means of improving the outcome for patients with rectal cancer, they are essential.

Having looked at technique and its effects in rectal cancer surgery, the evidence relating to surgeon variability should therefore be examined.

## EVIDENCE FOR SURGEON VARIABILITY

The concept of surgeon-related variability in the treatment of colorectal cancer was first formally recognized in the large bowel cancer project.[39] This study was based on 4228 patients treated by

94 surgeons in 23 hospitals in the United Kingdom, between 1974 and 1980. Overall, the incidence of anastomotic leakage was 13% but varied from 0.5% to over 30% depending on the senior surgeon responsible for the patient's care. Leakage was more common after anterior resection than after other colonic operations but did not account for the variability.[40] Local recurrence after apparently curative operations was found to vary from less than 5% to over 20% among surgeons entering 30 patients or more into the study.[41]

Another important early study in 1991 by McArdle and Hole[42] reported the results in 645 consecutive patients managed by 13 consultant surgeons between 1974 and 1979. After apparently curative resection, postoperative mortality varied from 0 to 20% and the anastomotic dehiscence rate from 0 to 25%. Locoregional recurrence varied from 0 to 21% and the 10-year survival rate from 20 to 63%. A multivariate analysis identified age, sex, emergency admission, Dukes' stage, and pre-existing cardiac or respiratory disease as risk factors predicting postoperative mortality. On the basis of these factors, adjusted hazard rate ratio for each of the surgeons were calculated and the variation was found to be 0.56–2.03%.[42]

Both of these studies provide fairly convincing evidence of surgeon-related variation but it must be emphasized that they represent surgical practice over 20 years ago and very few of the surgeons in these studies could have been regarded as colorectal cancer specialists. There is good evidence that overall results have changed and in the recent comprehensive population-based study carried out in the Wales and Trent region, the overall anastomotic dehiscence rate after anterior resection was only 5%.[17]

More recently, in the German audit of rectal cancer surgeons, 594 patients undergoing apparently curative resection between 1984 and 1986 were studied.[10] There were 14 surgeons responsible for more than 15 operations in the time period of the study. The 5-year survival of their patients varied between 40 and 80%. Likewise, the rate of locoregional recurrence varied from 4 to 55% and multiple logistic regression analysis showed that the individual surgeon was an independent risk factor for local recurrence. In the Edinburgh and Lothians large bowel cancer project 750 consecutive patients were treated between 1990 and 1992, and there were 28 different surgeons involved. The proportion of patients with rectal cancer in whom an anastomosis was achieved varied from 40 to 100% and the anastomotic dehiscence rate varied from 0 to 75%. Even when only the high-volume surgeons were studied, wide variations were seen.[43]

Thus, even with relatively contemporary studies, there is good evidence of variability in outcome which can be attributed to the individual surgeon. However, the problem of how to identify a surgeon who is likely to obtain good outcomes in rectal cancer surgery remains unsolved. One of the most obvious parameters is case volume and indeed the recent study from the Wales and Trent region showed that in the United Kingdom the number of patients with colorectal cancer treated by individual surgeons varied from 1 to 98 in a one year period.[17]

## Evidence for the effect of case volume

As far as the effect of case volume on outcome following colorectal cancer surgery is concerned, the evidence is conflicting. In the large bowel cancer project the incidence of anastomotic dehiscence was independent of the number of anastomoses performed (under 10 cases, 12.3%; 10–19 cases, 13.7%; 20 or more cases, 12.8%).[40] Likewise, McArdle & Hole[42] were unable to demonstrate any variation in outcome related to case volume. In their study the number of cases supervised by the individual surgeons varied from 21 to 98 over the period of study but this did not relate to curative resection rate, postoperative morbidity, or postoperative mortality, even when adjusted for the significant risk factors. It must be appreciated, however, that in both of these studies the surgeons examined were not necessarily the operating surgeons and it is likely that a substantial proportion of the patients were operated on by trainees who may or may not have been supervised.

In the rectal cancer study from Germany, the outcomes for 14 high-volume surgeons who had performed 15 or more rectal resections were compared with those for a group of low-volume surgeons.[44] A multivariate analysis including the stage of the tumor, the grade of the tumor, and the type of operation, revealed that there were three groups with significantly different rates of local recurrence. There was a single high-volume surgeon with a high local recurrence rate, there was a group of low-volume surgeons who had an intermediate rate, and all the other high-volume surgeons had the lowest rate. Thus, with a single exception, the high-volume surgeons obtained better results than the low-volume surgeons. In Lothian and Borders, it was found that of the 28 surgeons studied, only five were responsible for 50% of the rectal cancer patients and the anastomotic leak rate amongst these high-volume surgeons was lower when compared with the others.[43] In the audit from the Wales and Trent region, there was no association found between case volume for elective rectal cancer surgery and operative mortality, permanent stoma rate, anastomotic dehiscence or 3-year local recurrence and survival rates.[17]

Despite these equivocal findings, a recent careful study from Canada has demonstrated a marked case volume effect.[45] In this study, 683 rectal cancer patients treated by 52 surgeons were studied; 5-year follow up was available for 98% of the subjects. Multivariate analysis demonstrated that the surgeons performing less than 21 resections over the 8-year study period were significantly more likely to experience local recurrence (hazard ratio 1.8, $P=0.001$) and had a significantly higher disease-specific mortality rate (hazard ratio 1.4, $P=0.0005$).

Thus it would appear that although case volume may have an effect, it is difficult to demonstrate and the evidence is far from clear. The other approach for trying to identify factors that determine surgeon-related variability is to look at specialization, and this is dealt with in the next section.

## The effect of specialization

Perhaps the most obvious indication of an effect of specialization in rectal cancer surgery comes from the results of the individuals who practice TME (see above). However, although the results of these particular individuals can be regarded as 'gold standards,' some commentators believe that their results may be explained at least in part by selection of relatively favorable cases.[46] To obtain a more objective view of specialization, there are a number of large-scale studies, particularly from Sweden, which provide useful information. In the Swedish county of Ostergotland all patients with rectal cancer were treated by one of eight surgeons who used the technique of total mesorectal excision from 1989 onwards.[7] Adjuvant chemotherapy was not used at all and adjuvant radiotherapy was used only in four patients. In order to evaluate this strategy, a group of 211 cases treated between 1984 and 1986 was compared with a group of 230 treated between 1990 and 1992. Actuarial analysis revealed a significant reduction in local recurrence and a significant increase in crude survival rate in the group treated after the introduction of specialization.

In Uppsala, Sweden, it was possible to conduct a similar study owing to concentration of all rectal cancer surgery in a university colorectal unit in 1980.[47] The regular use of preoperative adjuvant radiotherapy was initiated at the same time and the routine employment of TME was started in 1985. All registered rectal cancer patients in Sweden between 1960 and 1989 were studied and although the 5-year survival steadily improved throughout the country this trend was more pronounced in Uppsala and particularly in the period between 1985 and 1989. It is interesting to note that patients with carcinoma of the colon had a better prognosis than those with carcinoma of the rectum, except in Uppsala between 1985 and 1989 where the reverse was the case. This study provides a strong argument for TME as it would appear that with careful surgery, cure rates for rectal cancer can be higher than those rates achieved for colonic cancer. As part of the same study, local recurrence rates were also studied and it was found that in the period 1974–1979 a local recurrence rate of 47% was recorded. Between 1980 and 1984 (after the introduction of adjuvant preoperative radiotherapy) this fell to 13% and after the introduction of TME in 1985 it fell to 11%.[47]

As part of the Stockholm trials of preoperative radiotherapy, local recurrence rate and death from rectal cancer were studied in 1399 patients.[48] The local recurrence was less when patients were treated by certified specialists of at least 10 years' standing (relative risk 0.8). A similar finding was reported for death from rectal cancer. In the Canadian study[45] a colorectal surgeon was defined as an individual who had held a post general colorectal training fellowship. The outcome results from the cohort of 683 patients were analyzed according to whether or not the patient had been treated by one of these colorectal specialists. There were only five such surgeons among the 52 surgeons studied, but they performed 16% of the operations. Again, using multivariate analysis the risk of developing local recurrence was found to be greater among the patients of surgeons who had not been trained in colorectal surgery (hazard ratio 2.5, $P = 0.001$). Furthermore, increased disease-specific mortality was seen with the noncolorectal trained surgeons (hazard ratio 1.5, $P = 0.001$).

A similar assessment was performed of 448 surgeons in South Florida. Three groups were included in the statewide database:[49] surgeons certified by the American Board of Colon and Rectal Surgery (ABCRS) in academic practice in teaching programs accredited by the accreditation council; surgeons certified by the

ABCRS but not faculty in colorectal training programs; and surgeons not certified by the ABCRS. The relationship found was from the first group to the third, a decrease in volume and an increase in cost despite stratification for severity of illness. Thus, not only does colorectal specialization predict better rates of recurrence, but they can be achieved at lower cost.

## CONCLUSIONS

From the available evidence, there is little doubt that the surgeon can influence the outcome in rectal cancer surgery both in terms of disease control and functional results. For the former variable at least, there is good evidence that a policy of specialization improves outcomes; isolated case volume has not been shown to be of significance, but this finding is not surprising as no amount of experience will be of value if appropriate training and expertise are lacking. The challenge for the future is to ensure that all surgeons dealing with rectal cancer are properly trained, and for this important goal to be achieved a system of accreditation that assesses technical proficiency in the relevant operative procedures is necessary. Periodic recertification may also play a role.

## REFERENCES

1    MRCRCWP (Medical Research Council Rectal Cancer Working Party). Randomised trial of surgery alone versus radiotherapy followed by surgery for potentially operable locally advanced rectal cancer. *Lancet* 1996;**348**:1605–1610

2    SRCT (Swedish Rectal Cancer Trial). Improved survival with pre-operative radiotherapy in resectable rectal cancer. *N Engl J Med* 1997;**336**:980–987

3    MRCRCWP (Medical Research Council Rectal Cancer Working Party). Randomised trial of surgery alone versus surgery followed by radiotherapy for mobile cancer of the rectum. *Lancet* 1996;**348**:1610–1614

4    McFarlane JK, Ryall RDH, Heald RJ. Mesorectal excision for rectal cancer. *Lancet* 1993;**341**:457–460

5    Enker WE, Thaler HT, Cranor ML, Polyak T. Total mesorectal excision in the operative treatment of carcinoma of the rectum. *J Am Coll Surg* 1995;**181**:335–346

6    Singh S, Morgan MBF, Broughton M, Caffarey S, Topham C, Marks CG. A ten-year prospective audit of outcome of surgical treatment for colorectal carcinoma. *Br J Surg* 1995;**82**:1486–1490

7    Arbman G, Nilsson E, Hallbook O, Sjodahl R. Local recurrence following total mesorectal excision for rectal cancer. *Br J Surg* 1996;**83**:375–379

8    Aitken RJ. Mesorectal excision for rectal cancer. *Br J Surg* 1996;**83**:214–216

9    Abulafi AM, Williams NS. Local recurrence of colorectal cancer: the problem, mechanisms, management and adjuvant therapy. *Br J Surg* 1994;**81**:7–19

10   Hermanek P, Wiebelt H, Staimmer D, Riedl S and the German Study Group for Colorectal Cancer. Prognostic factors of rectum carcinoma – experience of the German multicentre study SGCRC. *Tumori* 1995;**81**(suppl):60–64

11   Adam IJ, Mohamadee MO, Martin IG *et al*. Role of circumferential margin involvement in the local recurrence of rectal cancer. *Lancet* 1994;**344**:707–711

12   Scott N, Jackson P, Al-Jaberi T, Dixon MF, Quirke P, Finan PJ. Total mesorectal excision and local recurrence: a study of tumour spread in the mesorectum distal to rectal cancer. *Br J Surg* 1995;**82**:1031–1033

13   Heald RJ, Goligher JC. Anterior resection of the rectum. In: Fielding LP, Goldberg SM (eds) *Surgery of the Colon, Rectum and Anus (Rob and Smith's Operative Surgery)*, 5th edn. Butterworth Heinemann, London, pp 456–471

14   Hainsworth PJ, Egan MJ, Cunliffe WJ. Evaluation of a policy of total mesorectal excision for rectal and rectosigmoid cancers. *Br J Surg* 1997;**84**:652–656

15   Karanjia ND, Corder AP, Bearn P, Heald RJ. Leakage from stapled low anastomosis after total mesorectal excision of carcinoma of the rectum. *Br J Surg* 1994;**81**: 1224–1226

16   Carlsen E, Schlichting E, Guldvog I, Johnson E, Heald RJ. Effect of introduction of total mesorectal excision for the treatment of rectal cancer. *Br J Surg* 1998;**85**: 526–529

17   Mella J, Biffin A, Radcliffe AG, Stamatakis JD, Steele RJC. Population-based audit of colorectal management in two UK health regions. *Br J Surg* 1997;**84**: 1731–1736

18   Matheson NA, McIntosh CA, Krukowski ZH. Continuing experience with single layer appositional anastomosis in the large bowel. *Br J Surg* 1985(suppl): S104–S106

19   Moriya Y, Hojo K, Sawanda T, Koyama Y. Significance of lateral node dissection for advanced rectal carcinoma at or below the peritoneal reflection. *Dis Colon Rectum* 1989;**23**:307–315

20   Maas CP, Moriya Y, Steup WH *et al*. Radical and nerve-preserving surgery for rectal cancer in the Netherlands: a prospective study on morbidity and functional outcome. *Br J Surg* 1998;**85**:92–97

21   Camilleri-Brennan J, Steele RJC. Quality of life after treatment for rectal cancer. *Br J Surg* 1998;**85**:1036–1043

22   Ortiz H, Armendariz P. Anterior resection: do the patients perceive any clinical benefit? *Int J Colorectal Dis* 1996;**11**:191–195

23   Williams NS, Dixon MF, Johnston D. Reappraisal of the 5 cm rule of distal excision for carcinoma of the rectum: a study of distal intramural spread and of patients' survival. *Br J Surg* 1983;**70**:150–154

24   Karanjia ND, Schache DJ, North WR, Heald RJ. 'Close shave' in anterior resection. *Br J Surg* 1990;**77**:510–512

25   Lazorthes F, Fages P, Chiotasso P, Lemozy J, Bloom E. Resection of the rectum with construction of a colonic reservoir and colo-anal anastomosis for carcinoma of the rectum. *Br J Surg* 1986;**73**:136–138

26 Ortiz H, De Miguel M, Armendariz P, Rodriguez J, Chocarro C. Colo-anal anastomosis: are functional results better with a pouch? *Dis Colon Rectum* 1995;38:375–377

27 Hallbook O, Pahlman I, Krog M, Wexner SD, Sjodahl R. Randomised comparison of straight and colonic J-pouch anastomosis after low anterior resection. *Ann Surg* 1996;224:58–65

28 Ho YH, Tan M, Seow-Choen F. Prospective randomised controlled study of clinical function and anorectal physiology after low anterior resection: comparison of straight and colonic J-pouch anastomosis. *Br J Surg* 1996;83:978–980

29 Parc R, Tiret E, Frilauxoszkowski E, Loygue J. Resection and colo-anal anastomosis with colonic reservoir for rectal carcinoma. *Br J Surg* 1986;73:139–141

30 Hida J, Yasutomi M, Fujimoto K *et al.* Functional outcome after low anterior resection with low anastomosis for rectal cancer using the colonic J-pouch. Prospective randomised study for determination of optimum pouch size. *Dis Colon Rectum* 1996;39:986–991

31 Banerjee AK, Jehle EC, Shorthouse AJ, Buess G. Local excision of rectal tumours. *Br J Surg* 1995;82:1165–1173

32 Blumberg D, Paty PB, Gullem JG *et al.* All patients with small intramural rectal cancers are at risk for lymph node metastases. *Dis Colon Rectum* 1999;42:881–885

33 Killingback M. Local excision of carcinoma of the rectum: indications. *World J Surg* 1992;16:437–446

34 Hermanek P, Marzoli GP. *Local Therapy of Rectum Carcinoma*. Springer, Berlin, 1994

35 Winde G, Nottberg H, Keller R, Schmid KW, Bunte H. Surgical cure for early rectal carcinomas (T1). *Dis Colon Rectum* 1996;39:969–976

36 Le Voyer TE, Hoffman JP, Cooper H, Ross E, Sigurdson E, Eisenberg B. Local excision and chemoradiation for low rectal T1 and T2 cancers is an effective treatment. *Am Surg* 1999;65;625–630

37 Wagman R, Minsky BD, Cohen AM, Saltz L, Paty PB, Guillem JG. Conservative management of rectal cancer with local excision and postoperative adjuvant therapy. *Int J Radiat Oncol Biol Phys* 1999;44:841–846

38 Lezoche E, Guerrieri M, Paganini AM, Feliciotti F. Transanal endoscopic microsurgical excision of irradiated and nonirradiated rectal cancer. A 5-year experience. *Surg Laparosc Endosc* 1998;8:249–256

39 Fielding LP, Stewart-Brown S, Dudley HAF. Surgeon-related variables and the clinical trial. *Lancet* 1978;2:778–779

40 Fielding LP, Stewart-Brown S, Blesovsky L, Kearney G. Anastomotic integrity after operations for large-bowel cancer: a multicentre study. *Br Med J* 1980;281:411–414

41 Phillips RKS, Hittinger R, Blesovsky L, Fry JS, Fielding LP. Local recurrence following 'curative' surgery for large bowel cancer: I. The overall picture. *Br J Surg* 1984;71:12–16

42 McArdle CS, Hole D. Impact of variability among surgeons on postoperative morbidity and mortality and ultimate survival. *Br Med J* 1991;302:1501–1505

43  Carter DC for the consultant surgeons and pathologists of the Lothian and Borders Health Boards. Lothian and Borders large bowel cancer project: immediate outcome after surgery. *Br J Surg* 1995;**82**:888–890

44  Hermanek P, Hohenberger W. The importance of volume in colorectal cancer surgery. *Eur J Surg Oncol* 1996;**22**:213–215

45  Porter GA, Soskolne CL, Yakimets WW, Newman SC. Surgeon-related factors and outcome in rectal cancer. *Ann Surg* 1998;**227**:157–167

46  Scholefield JH, Northover JMA. Surgical management of rectal cancer. *Br J Surg* 1995;**82**:745–748

47  Dahlberg M, Glimelius B, Pahlman L. Changing strategy for rectal cancer is associated with improved outcome. *Br J Surg* 1999;**86**:379–384

48  Holm T, Johansson H, Cedermark B, Ekelund G, Rutqvist LE. Influence of hospital- and surgeon-related factors on outcome after treatment of rectal cancer with or without preoperative radiotherapy. *Br J Surg* 1997;**84**:657–663

49  Latulippe JF, Potenti F, Weiss E, Nogueras JJ, Wexner SD. Impact of colorectal board certification and volume: charges of colon and rectal surgery (abstract). *Dis Colon Rectum* 1998;**41**:A53

# Why is preoperative better than postoperative radiotherapy?

*Lars Påhlman*

## INTRODUCTION

The rationale of radiotherapy, sometimes in combination with chemotherapy, in the management of patients with primary rectal cancer is defined in two main groups of patients. For those patients with a fixed rectal cancer, i.e. large $T_3$ or a $T_4$ cancer, more or less 'non-resectable' rectal cancer, the role of preoperative irradiation will not be discussed, since today there is no controversy on this line of management, and it is considered almost negligent not to prescribe radiotherapy with or without a combination of chemotherapy in these patients. This chapter focuses on the role of either pre- or postoperative radiotherapy, with or without chemotherapy, in the treatment of resectable rectal cancer (stages $T_1$–$T_3$). This is, by definition, adjuvant treatment, and its value is still being debated. In this group of patients the objective is to eradicate micrometastases outside the surgical plane of dissection in order to reduce the often unacceptable high local recurrence rate and consequently improve the overall survival.

## IS ADJUVANT RADIOTHERAPY REQUIRED?

Surgery remains the most essential component of the treatment of rectal cancer although its main drawback is a rather high local recurrence rate as reported in some series. The local recurrence rates have varied considerably from less than 5% up to 50%.[1,2] It is difficult to explain this discrepancy, but possible explanations for this may be the differences in data analyses, follow-up policies, definition of radicality, and patient selection, but probably most important is the surgeon's skill. According to several randomized trials the average recurrence rate is 25% after surgery alone compared with less than 20% when surgery is combined with pre- or postoperative radiotherapy. These figures probably reflect the results of standard surgery in rectal cancer. When institutions have reported less than a 10% local recurrence rate, this was attributed by the critics to patient selection rather than to the operative group.[1,3] However, adopting lymph node clearance in order to reduce local recurrence[4] has been associated with postoperative morbidity, particularly sexual and bladder dysfunction.[5] An important question is whether local recurrence has an impact on survival; this has been addressed directly. In one series from Germany, it was found that surgeons with high local recurrence rates had a worse 5-year survival among their patients, compared with surgeons with low local recurrence rates.[6]

The rationale of adjuvant radiotherapy is ideal since radiotherapy is mainly effective in the periphery of the tumor, where tumor cell size is limited and the area is well vascularized and oxygenated. The surgeon debulks the tumor mass, preserving the normal tissue adjacent to the tumor where irradiation is given to this area that may contain tumor deposits not recognizable by the surgeon. Whether chemotherapy has an impact on the local control is still unclear but there are some data indicating that chemotherapy will even enhance the effect of radiotherapy.

## PATIENT SELECTION

The most important task for surgeons managing rectal cancer is the evaluation of its resectability. If a tumor is considered fixed and non-mobile, which means a large bulky $T_3$ or $T_4$ tumor, the patient should be submitted to preoperative radiotherapy to achieve tumor shrinkage and if possible make the surgical attempt curative. The evaluation of fixity can sometimes be difficult but is facilitated with an examination under anesthesia and computed tomography or magnetic resonance imaging.

Patients who are usually considered for adjuvant treatment are those with a mobile tumor. In this group of patients endoanal ultrasonography is the preferable method to evaluate the extent of tumor growth through the bowel wall (muscularis propria). While the benefit of radiotherapy in patients with $T_1$ and $T_2$ tumors is arguable, the evidence indicates that in $T_3$ tumors radiotherapy is necessary.

## ADJUVANT RADIOTHERAPY

### Pre- or postoperative?

Radiotherapy has been given pre- or postoperatively for many decades in rectal cancer as an additional treatment modality and both options have been evaluated in randomized trials. The pros and cons of either treatment with respect to efficacy (reduction of the local recurrence rate) and morbidity are summarized in Table 11.1 and are discussed in detail below.

### Irradiation technique

There is difficulty in evaluating the results in most trials reported in the literature because of differences in dose levels, fractionation schedules, and target volumes. The rationale for using different

**Table 11.1** Advantages and disadvantages of pre- and postoperative irradiation

|  | Preoperative irradiation | Postoperative irradiation |
|---|---|---|
| Reduction of local tumor, increasing resectability | Yes | No |
| Delay in administering irradiation due to wound healing | No | Yes |
| Hypoxic cells in the periphery of the tumors at irradiation – reducing radiosensitivity | No | Yes |
| Tumor cell repopulation | No | Yes |
| Reduced circulating viable tumor cells at surgery | Yes | No |
| With postoperative adhesions, small bowel may be at greater risk | No | Yes |
| Dukes' A lesions excluded | No | Yes |
| Patients with distant metastases can be excluded | No | Yes |
| Surgery delayed | Yes | No |
| Influence on wound healing | Yes | No |

techniques has been presented elsewhere.[6] Briefly, the dose has to be sufficiently high to destroy micrometastases with acceptable probability. The minimum dose required to destroy a micrometastasis (less than a few millimeters in diameter, at most $10^8$ cells) with a high probability is about 45 gray (Gy) given in 5 weeks. This dose can be reached with different fractionation schedules, and the method used in Sweden, $5 \times 5$ Gy in 1 week, is equivalent to a dose of 50 Gy given during a 5-week period with conventional fractionation.

In order to compare the dose regimens used in different trials it is important to estimate the biological effect of the irradiation. The reason for this is that the radiation effect is not only dependent on the total dose but also the dose at each fraction and overall treatment time. Therefore, all trials using pre- or postoperative radiotherapy have been compiled in Table 11.2 according the biological effect of radiation using the linear quadratic (LQ) time formula.[7]

## Effect on local recurrence rates

Since the required dose to kill micrometastases with a high probability corresponds to an LQ time about 45 Gy, no effect on local recurrence rates has been demonstrated in trials where considerably lower doses (LQ time $< 25$ Gy) have been employed. Furthermore, two dominating observations can be drawn out from the results listed in the table. First, there is a clear dose–response relationship and reduction in local recurrence rates; and, secondly, the reduction in local recurrence rate at a given dose was higher in the trials where preoperative irradiation was given, indicating that preoperative radiotherapy is more dose-effective than postoperative irradiation.

An important factor is the fractionation schedule. Normally 1.8–2 Gy fraction has been used, and even with such a conventional fractionation in a preoperative setting, which is a moderate dose (LQ time 26.8–35.2), the local recurrence rate is reduced.[12,14] A more time-sparing treatment schedule, with 5 Gy fractions, has also been used with different numbers of fractions. In the five trials where 5 Gy fractions were used, a clear dose–response relationship is observed dependent upon the numbers of fractions given per week.[8–10,18,19] At least $3 \times 5$ Gy[10] or preferably $5 \times 5$ Gy[18,19] has to be used. In the largest trial, the Swedish Rectal Cancer Trial, the local recurrence rate in the surgery alone group was 27% compared with 11% in the irradiated group, giving a relative reduction in the local recurrence rate of 61%.[19]

**Table 11.2** Pelvic recurrence after a combination of surgery and radiotherapy in rectal carcinoma (controlled trials with a surgery alone group)

| Study (reference no.) | Irradiation dose (Gy)/no. of fractions | LQ time | Surgery alone | | Surgery + radiotherapy | | P value[a] | Percent reduction in local failure rates |
|---|---|---|---|---|---|---|---|---|
| | | | No. of local recurrences/ total | % | No. of local recurrences/ total | % | | |
| *Preoperative* | | | | | | | | |
| Toronto[8] | 5/1 | 7.5 | b | | | | | |
| MRC I[9] | 5/1 | 7.5 | c | | | | | |
| | 20/10 | 20.4 | c | | | | | |
| St Marks[10] | 15/3 | 22.5 | 51/210 | 24 | 31/185 | 17 | * | 29 |
| VASOG II[11] | 31.5/18 | 26.8 | b | | | | | |
| Bergen[12] | 31.5/18 | 26.8 | 31/131 | 24 | 24/138 | 17 | NS | 29 |
| VASOG I[13] | 25/10 | 27.5 | 32/87 | 37 | 27/93 | 22 | NS | 22 |
| North-West[14] | 20/4 | 30.0 | 46/126 | 37 | 17/133 | 13 | ** | 65 |
| EORTC[15] | 34.5/15 | 35.2 | 49/175 | 28 | 24/166 | 14 | ** | 50 |
| Brazil[16] | 40/20 | 36.0 | 17/36 | 47 | 5/32 | 15 | ** | 63 |

| | | | | | | | |
|---|---|---|---|---|---|---|---|
| MRC 2[17d] | 40/20 | 36.0 | 65/140 | 46 | 50/129 | 36 | * | 22 |
| SRCSG[18] | 25/5 | 37.5 | 120/425 | 28 | 61/424 | 14 | *** | 50 |
| SRCT[19] | 25/5 | 37.5 | 150/557 | 27 | 63/553 | 11 | *** | 60 |
| *Postoperative* | | | | | | | |
| Odense[20] | 50/25 | 35.4 | 57/250 | 23 | 46/244 | 19 | NS | 174 |
| MRC 3[21] | 40/20 | 36.0 | 74/235 | 34 | 48/234 | 21 | ** | 38 |
| GITSG[22] | 40–48/22 | 36.0 | 27/106 | 25 | 15/96 | 16 | NS | 36 |
| NSABP[23] | 46.5/26 | 39.3 | 45/184 | 24 | 30/184 | 16 | NS | 33 |
| EORTC[24] | 46/23 | 40.8 | 30/88 | 34 | 25/84 | 30 | NS | 13 |
| Rotterdam[25] | 50/25 | 43.8 | 28/84 | 33 | 21/88 | 24 | NS | 41 |

[a] NS = $P > 0.05$, * = $P < 0.05$, ** = $P < 0.01$, *** = $P < 0.001$.

[b] Not reported.

[c] Only actuarial data reported, with no difference between groups.

[d] Only tethered tumors.

Postoperative radiotherapy is not as effective as preoperative irradiation, although the dose has been 15–20 Gy higher in the trials where postoperative irradiation has been given. Even with a dose of 50 Gy (LQ time 35.4–43.8), there was no significant reduction in the local recurrence rate,[20,22–25] but when postoperative radiotherapy was combined with chemotherapy the effect on the local failure rates was improved but not to the same magnitude as with preoperative regimens.[22,23] Only one trial using postoperative radiotherapy (40 Gy was given in 4 weeks) has shown a significant reduction,[21] and another trial (50 Gy in 25 fractions) has shown a tendency toward a reduction in local recurrence rates.[25]

Only one trial, the Uppsala trial in Sweden, has compared pre- and postoperative radiotherapy in which patients were randomly allocated to receive either preoperative or postoperative radiotherapy.[26,27] In the preoperative group 25.5 Gy was given in five fractions of 5.1 Gy daily over a 5–7 day period (CRE 14.0, LQ time 38.0) followed by surgery the week after. In the postoperative group only patients with Dukes' stage B or C received radiotherapy. Irradiation commenced within 6 weeks and was given in 2 Gy daily fractions, 5 days a week for 4–5 weeks, with a split of 10–14 days after 40 Gy and further irradiation was given for a period of 2 weeks, up to a total dose of 60 Gy (CRE 16.9, LQ time 46.9). Although this was the highest dose ever used as an adjuvant postoperative treatment, the local recurrence rate after a minimum of 5 years' follow up was lower in the preoperatively irradiated group (12%) than in the postoperative group (21%) ($P<0.02$).[26]

In summary, all available data indicate that preoperative irradiation is more dose-effective than postoperative irradiation in reducing the local recurrence rates. Two possible explanations for the higher efficacy of preoperative radiotherapy are the repopulation of tumor cells after surgery (the cells to be destroyed are simply more numerous after than before surgery), and/or, the cells to be destroyed in the infiltrating zones are better oxygenated before surgery.

## Influence on survival

### Radiotherapy alone

In a meta-analysis including all controlled trials published up to 1984, a marginal improvement of survival by 4.3% was noted in the irradiated group of patients.[28] This is not easy to explain since radiotherapy to the primary tumor bed does not affect occult distant metastases. However, in at least 20% of all patients resected for cure, local failure is the only sign of residual tumor. Therefore, it is conceivable that radiotherapy will have an indirect impact on survival with prolonged follow up provided the local recurrence rate is reduced.

In the meta-analysis described, trials using moderate to high dose radiotherapy were not included: namely, the North-West[14] and the Imperial Cancer Research Fund trials in England,[10] and the Swedish Rectal Cancer Trial.[19] The latter trial was designed to detect a survival benefit of 10% with the hypothesis that the local recurrence rate could be halved. After a minimum of 5 years' follow up a statistically significant overall survival benefit (48% vs 58%) was found in the group of patients who received 1-week preoperative radiotherapy ($5 \times 5$ Gy).[19] No effect on survival has been demonstrated in the trials where postoperative radiotherapy alone has been used.[20,21,23–25] However, there was no survival difference between preoperative and postoperative radiotherapy in the Uppsala trial.[26]

## Combination with chemotherapy

The concept of combining radiotherapy with chemotherapy has some theoretical advantages,[29,30] and has been adopted in the United States where chemotherapy is combined with postoperative radiotherapy. In the Gastrointestinal Tumour Study Group (GITSG) trial, a survival benefit was noticed in the group of patients who received both radiotherapy and chemotherapy.[22] In the National Surgical Adjuvant Breast and Colorectal Project (NSABP) trial, postoperative radiotherapy had no effect on survival, whereas chemotherapy alone improved survival when compared with surgery alone.[23] In the North Central Cancer Treatment Group (NCCTG) trial, postoperative radiotherapy alone was compared with postoperative chemo–radiotherapy and an improved survival was found in the combined group.[31] Based on the results in these three American trials, the Consensus Conference of the National Institute of Health in the United States recommended that standard treatment for patients with a tumor in Dukes' stage B or C should be postoperative adjuvant chemo–radiotherapy.[32] A recently published Norwegian controlled randomized trial where patients received postoperative radio-therapy (46 Gy, CRE 14.9, LQ time 39.3) combined with 5-FU (5-fluorouracil), showed a reduction in the local recurrence rate of 50%, and this reduction had an impact on overall survival.[33]

The survival improvement observed in the Swedish Rectal Cancer Trial is of the same magnitude as that reported in the American and Norwegian postoperative combined chemo–radiotherapy trials. Since preoperative radiotherapy is more dose-effective than postoperative radiotherapy, it might be possible that the survival benefit reported in the other mentioned trials is attributed to a chemotherapy effect, since patients allocated to the chemo–radiotherapy arm continued on chemotherapy for 1 year in some trials. According to available data, it seems logical to give the patients preoperative radiotherapy and to add chemotherapy postoperatively in those with more advanced cancer, i.e. tumors in stages II or III. No trial has used preoperative chemo–radiotherapy in an adjuvant setting, but one German, one French, and two American trials are ongoing where preoperative chemo–radiotherapy is tested against postoperative chemo–radiotherapy.

## Is adjuvant radiotherapy safe?

Overtreatment is the main concern when adjuvant treatment is proposed and especially if preoperative irradiation is given to patients with a $T_1$ or $T_2$ tumor, i.e. a tumor in Dukes' stage A, or patients with disseminated disease found at surgery. Although it is possible to identify Dukes' A lesions with preoperative endoanal ultrasound examination of the rectum, it is important to reduce morbidity by careful clinical staging preoperatively.

### Postoperative mortality

An increase in postoperative mortality has been observed after preoperative irradiation and has been reported in the Stockholm-Malmö and St Mark's Hospital trials among elderly patients (above 75 years of age) and in those with disseminated disease discovered at surgery. This was not the experience in the Uppsala trial, although the same dose was used as in the Stockholm-Malmö trial. However, different irradiation techniques were used (three fields in Uppsala; multiple fields in the North West trial) to avoid irradiation of those parts of the pelvis and abdomen that should not be included in the target. The difference in postoperative mortality between Stockholm and Uppsala was one important reason why the Swedish Rectal Cancer trial ($5 \times 5$ Gy in 1 week) was undertaken, in which postoperative mortality was one of the main end points. According to the protocol, the use of three or four portals was mandatory. In four hospitals where the two-portal technique was used, postoperative mortality was increased significantly.[34] However, no difference in hospital mortality was found in the surgery alone arm or among the patients irradiated with a three- or four-portal technique (2.6% vs 2.6%), indicating that preoperative high-dose short-course radiotherapy could be administered safely without increasing postoperative mortality.[34]

### Postoperative morbidity

The risk of a perineal wound infection after an abdominoperineal excision is increased from 10% to 20% when preoperative radiotherapy is given.[26,34,35] Conversely, a chronic perineal sinus is not more frequent when radiotherapy has been given.[27] No increase in postoperative abdominal wound, pulmonary, or urinary infection has been reported after preoperative irradiation in the controlled trials. Furthermore, experimental data indicate that preoperative radiotherapy does not interfere with anastomotic healing[36] and in all controlled randomized trials[10,14,15,18,19] subsequently no increase in anastomotic dehiscence has been observed after preoperative radiotherapy.

### Tolerance to treatment

If radiotherapy is used it is important that patients receive the planned treatment. By definition, preoperative treatment would have more or less a 100% compliance, whereas this would be less for postoperative irradiation, mainly due to prolonged postoperative recovery but also due to radiotherapy complications. In the Uppsala trial, acute adverse effects to pre- and postoperative radiotherapy were prospectively recorded. Preoperative treatment was well tolerated and the compliance was 99.6% (only one of the patients who were allocated to preoperative irradiation did not receive the treatment), in contrast to postoperative irradiation which was completed without any complications in only 9% of the patients.[37] The problem with compliance has also been reported in the AXIS-trial in the UK, where 96% of patients in the preoperative arm received the treatment compared with 58% in the postoperative group (AXIS Trial Centre, personal communication). Also, similar difficulties were reported in the Danish trial using postoperative radiotherapy where only 85% of the patients who started the postoperative irradiation completed the treatment.[20]

If postoperative chemo–radiotherapy is used, acute toxicity is even more pronounced, with chemotherapy-related side effects such as an increased risk of dermatitis in the irradiated area, diarrhea, and leukopenia.[22,23]

### Late adverse effects

Available data in the literature indicate that intestinal obstruction and change in bowel habits are not more common after preoperative radiotherapy than after surgery alone.[27,38] Although several techniques have been used to prevent the small bowel from descending into the lesser pelvis to minimize the risk of irradiation damage small bowel obstruction is a significantly common complication after postoperative radiotherapy.[20,27]

Other complications from areas within the target have been looked for extensively in a prospective study with independent re-examinations of all patients alive in the Uppsala trial. No specific late adverse effects were found in the preoperatively irradiated patients compared with those having surgery alone.[27] A similar review of all patients in the Stockholm trial showed an increased risk of venous thromboembolism, femoral neck or pelvic fractures, and fistulas among irradiated patients,[38] and the risk of late small bowel obstruction was clearly related to the size of the target.

Another concern after adjuvant radiotherapy is the anal sphincter function. After postoperative radiotherapy the sphincter function might be impaired[39] and data from the Swedish Rectal Cancer Trial indicate that preoperative radiotherapy also alters the sphincter function.[40]

## CONCLUSION

Due to a better dose–response effect in the reduction of the local recurrence rates, preoperative irradiation should be used if adjuvant radiotherapy is considered. With such a concept, patients with a $T_1$ or $T_2$ lesion and patients with metastatic disease have to be excluded. Using modern imaging techniques, this is not a problem.

A matter for consideration is that both pre- and postoperative radiotherapy have been evaluated in trials where surgery has not been 'optimized.' Since more 'optimized' surgery, as compared with so-called standard surgery, results in local failure rates similar to 'standard' surgery + radiotherapy[1,3,4] it can be argued that adjuvant radiotherapy is superfluous. This question is specifically addressed in a Dutch trial, which has recruited 1861 patients, where 'optimized' surgery is mandatory and where the patients are randomized either to receive or not receive preoperative ($5 \times 5$ Gy) radiotherapy. The study was closed in December 1999.

An important question is which type of fractionation schedule should be used, i.e. short-term, high-dose preoperative irradiation ($4–5 \times 5$ Gy) for 1 week or a more conventional fractionation ($25–30 \times 1.8–2.0$ Gy) for 5 weeks. The latter approach is more resource demanding. Another question is whether or not it is necessary to combine chemotherapy in order to further improve the outcome. This has not been examined in an adjuvant setting but trials are ongoing. Other important aspects of adjuvant radiotherapy are compliance and economic considerations, which support the use of preoperative radiotherapy.

## REFERENCES

1   MacFarlane JK, Ryall RD, Heald RJ. Mesorectal excision for rectal cancer. *Lancet* 1993;**341**:457–460

2   Gunderson LL, Sosin H. Areas of failure found at reoperation (second or symptomatic look) following 'curative surgery' for adenocarcinoma of the rectum. *Cancer* 1974;**34**:1278–1292

3   Enker WE, Laffer UT, Block GE. Enhanced survival of patients with colon and rectal cancer is based upon wide anatomic resection. *Ann Surg* 1979;**190**:350–360

4   Moriya Y, Hojo K, Sawada T, Koyama Y. Significance of lateral node dissection for advanced rectal carcinoma at or below the peritoneal reflection. *Dis Colon Rectum* 1989;**32**:307–315

5   Hojo K, Sawada T, Moroija Y. An analysis of survival and voiding, sexual function after wide iliopelvic lymphadenectomy in patients with carcinoma of the rectum, compared with conventional lymphadenectomy. *Dis Colon Rectum* 1989;**32**: 128–133

6   Glimelius B, Påhlman L. Perioperative radiotherapy in rectal cancer. *Acta Oncol* 1999;**38**:23–32

7   Fowler JF. The linear-quadratic formula and progress in fractionated radiotherapy. *Br J Radiol* 1989;**62**:679–694

8   Rider WD, Palmer JA, Mahoney L, Robertson CT. Preoperative irradiation in operable cancer of the rectum. *Can J Surg* 1977;**20**:335–338

9   Duncan W, Smith AN, Freedman LS *et al*. The evaluation of low dose pre-operative X-ray therapy in the management of operable rectal cancer; results of a randomly controlled trial. *Br J Surg* 1984;**71**:21–25

10 Goldberg PA, Nicholls RJ, Porter NH, Love S, Grimsey JE. Long-term results of a randomised trial of short-course low-dose adjuvant pre-operative radiotherapy for rectal cancer. Reduction in local treatment failure. *Eur J Cancer* 1994;**30A(11)**: 1602–1606

11 Higgins G, Humphrey E, Dwight R, Roswits B, Lee L, Keehn R. Preoperative radiation and surgery for cancer of the rectum. VASOG trial II. *Cancer* 1986;**58**:352–359

12 Horn A, Halvorsen JF, Dahl O. Preoperative radiotherapy in operable rectal cancer. *Dis Colon Rectum* 1990;**33**:823–828

13 Roswit B, Higgins G, Keehn R. Preoperative irradiation for carcinoma of the rectum and rectosigmoid colon: Report of a National Veterans Administration randomized study. *Cancer* 1975;**35**:1597–1602

14 James RD, Haboubi N, Schofield PF, Mellor M, Salhab N. Prognostic factors in colorectal carcinoma treated by preoperative radiotherapy and immediate surgery. *Dis Colon Rectum* 1991;**34**:546–551

15 Gérard A, Buyse M, Nordlinger B *et al*. Preoperative radiotherapy as adjuvant treatment in rectal cancer. *Ann Surg* 1988;**208**:606–614

16 Reis Neto JA, Quilici FA, Reis JA Jr. A comparison of nonoperative vs. preoperative radiotherapy in rectal carcinoma. A 10-years randomized trial. *Dis Colon Rectum* 1989;**32**:702–710

17 MRC 2 (Medical Research Council Rectal Cancer Working Party). Randomised trial of surgery alone versus radiotherapy followed by surgery for potentially operable locally advanced rectal cancer. *Lancet* 1996;**348**:1605–1610

18 SRCSG (Stockholm Rectal Cancer Study Group). Preoperative short-term radiation therapy in operable rectal carcinoma. *Cancer* 1990;**66**:49–53

19 SRCT (Swedish Rectal Cancer Trial). Improved survival with preoperative radiotherapy resectable rectal carcinoma. *N Engl J Med* 1997;**336**:980–987

20 Balslev I, Pedersen M, Teglbjaerg PS *et al*. Postoperative radiotherapy in Dukes' B and C carcinoma of the rectum and rectosigmoid. A randomized multicenter study. *Cancer* 1986;**58**:22–28

21 MRC 3 (Medical Research Council Rectal Cancer Working Party). Randomised trial of surgery alone versus surgery followed by radiotherapy for mobile cancer of the rectum. *Lancet* 1996;**348**:1610–1614

22 GITSG (Gastro Intestinal Tumour Study Group). Prolongation of the disease-free interval in surgically treated rectal carcinoma. *N Engl J Med* 1985;**312**:1464–1472

23 Fisher B, Wolmark N, Rockette H *et al*. Postoperative adjuvant chemotherapy or radiation therapy for rectal cancer: results from NSABP Protocol R-01. *JNCI* 1988;**80**:21–29

24 Arnaud JP, Nordlinger B, Bosset JF *et al*. Radical surgery and postoperative radiotherapy as combined treatment in rectal cancer. Final results of a phase III study of the European Organization for Research and Treatment of Cancer. *Br J Surg* 1997;**84**:352–357

25 Treuniet-Donker AD, van Putten WLJ. Postoperative radiation therapy for rectal cancer. *Cancer* 1991;**67**:2042–2048

26 Påhlman L, Glimelius B. Pre- and postoperative radiotherapy in rectal carcinoma: report from a randomized multicenter trial. *Ann Surg* 1990;**211**:187–195

27  Jansson-Frykholm G, Glimelius B, Påhlman L. Preoperative or postoperative irradiation in adenocarcinoma of the rectum: final treatment results of a randomized trial and an evaluation of late secondary effects. *Dis Colon Rectum* 1993;**36**: 564–572

28  Buyse M, Zeleniuch-Jacquotte A, Chalmers TC. Adjuvant therapy of colorectal cancer. Why we still don't know. *JAMA* 1988;**259**:3571–3578

29  Byfield J, Calabro-Jones P, Klisak I, Kulhanian F. Pharmacological requirements for obtaining sensitization of human tumor cells *in vitro* to combined 5-fluorouracil or Ftorafur and X-rays. *Int J Radiat Oncol Biol Phys* 1982;**8**:1923–1933

30  von der Maase H. Experimental studies on interactions of radiation and cancer chemotherapeutic drugs in normal tissues and a solid tumour. *Rad Oncol* 1986;**7**:47–68

31  Krook JE, Moertel CG, Gunderson LL *et al.* Effective surgical adjuvant therapy for high-risk rectal carcinoma. *N Eng J Med* 1991;**324**:709–715

32  NCI. Clinical announcement. Adjuvant therapy for rectal cancer. 1991;14 March

33  Tveit KM, Guldvog I, Hagen S *et al.* Randomized controlled trial of postoperative radiotherapy and short-term time-scheduled 5-fluorouracil against surgery alone in the treatment of Dukes' B and C rectal cancer. *Br J Surg* 1997;**84**:1130–1135

34  SRCT (Swedish Rectal Cancer Trial). Preoperative irradiation followed by surgery vs surgery alone in resectable rectal carcinoma – postoperative morbidity and mortality in a Swedish multicenter trial. *Br J Surg* 1993;**80**:1333–1336

35  Cedermark B, Johansson H, Rutquist LE, Wilking N. The Stockholm I trial of preoperative short term radiotherapy in operable rectal carcinoma. *Cancer* 1995;**75**:2269–2275

36  Bubrik MP, Rolfmeyers ES, Schauer RM *et al.* Effects of high-dose and low-dose preoperative irradiation on low anterior anastomosis in dogs. *Dis Colon Rectum* 1982;**25**:406–415

37  Påhlman L, Glimelius B, Graffman S. Pre- versus postoperative radiotherapy in rectal carcinoma: an interim report from a randomized multicentre trial. *Br J Surg* 1985;**72**:961–966

38  Holm T, Singnomklao T, Rutqvist L-E, Cedermark B. Adjuvant preoperative radiotherapy in patients with rectal carcinoma. Adverse effects during long term follow-up of two randomized trials. *Cancer* 1996;**78**:968–976

39  Lewis WG, Williamson MER, Kuzu A *et al.* Potential disadvantages of postoperative adjuvant radiotherapy after anterior resection for rectal cancer: a pilot study of sphincter function, rectal capacity and clinical outcome. *Int J Colorectal Dis* 1995;**10**:133–137

40  Dahlberg M, Glimelius B, Graf W, Påhlman L. Preoperative irradiation affects the functional results after surgery for rectal cancer: results from a randomized study. *Dis Colon Rectum* 1998;**41**:543–549

# 12 Can the irradiated rectum be preserved?

*Theodore J Saclarides and Marc I Brand*

Pelvic irradiation has an important role in the treatment of a variety of cancers of the genitourinary and gastrointestinal systems. Although the potential benefits of treatment are recognized, patients may experience distressing symptoms secondary to the treatment. Most gastrointestinal complications involve the rectum because of its fixed position in the pelvis and its close proximity to the treated area. Symptoms that arise because of these complications may be exacerbated if partial proctectomy is performed, thus reducing the capacity of the rectal reservoir. Rectal injuries may manifest as rectovaginal fistulas, anorectal strictures, or hemorrhagic proctitis. The small bowel may also be injured, however less commonly than the rectum. Small bowel injuries include obstruction, diarrhea and malabsorption, and fistulas to adjacent organs.

The focus of this chapter will be on the treatment of rectal complications of pelvic irradiation. The question as to whether the irradiated rectum can be saved depends on which specific complication is considered. Other factors, including patient age, presence of comorbidity, bowel function, rectal capacity and compliance, and anal sphincter function also enter into the decision-making process.

## INCIDENCE OF COMPLICATIONS

### Radiotherapy for prostate cancer

During pelvic radiotherapy virtually all patients experience some alteration in gastrointestinal function. Acute symptoms of bowel injury such as tenesmus, urgency, bleeding, diarrhea, and incontinence are common; such symptoms usually resolve within 2–3 months following the completion of radiation therapy. However, some patients will subsequently develop chronic problems. The technique and field of the potential for significant morbidity, proper patient selection for surgery is critical. A poor-risk patient might be better served with a well-constructed colostomy than a misplaced heroic effort at an extirpative reconstructive procedure.

Chronic hemorrhagic proctitis has been treated by a variety of means, most of which have been unsuccessful, including anti-inflammatory agents, topical steroid solutions, electrocautery, and laser ablation. When bleeding has persisted after these measures, surgeons have often resorted to fecal diversion as a means of treating chronic bleeding. Unfortunately, the bleeding often continues unabatedly. Various endoscopic laser modalities have emerged for the treatment of chronic radiation hemorrhagic proctitis; however, such forms of therapy are hampered by the fact that multiple endoscopic sessions are frequently necessary in order to produce any significant impact. Barbatzas et al.[20] reported nine patients who had previously undergone radiotherapy for pelvic cancer, a median of 14 months before the onset of rectal bleeding. Endoscopic ND:Yag laser treatment commenced a median of 4 months after the onset of blood loss and was repeated monthly until bleeding stopped; patients received an average of three laser treatments (range 1–5). Only one of the nine patients required transfusion after the completion of treatment, and in another six the bleeding was reduced to occasional spotting. Leuchter et al.[21] reported that four sessions were needed to control bleeding. The argon laser has also been used to control hemorrhagic proctitis. Taylor et al.[22] treated 14 patients with argon laser; a total of 51 procedures were performed, 71% of these needing 'maintenance' laser therapy. Therefore, although these laser modalities might seem attractive as a possible means to avoid surgery, they are unlikely to arrest the bleeding after a single session.

The instillation of formalin into the bladder was an accepted method of treating hemorrhagic radiation-induced cystitis. Initially, 10% concentrations were used; however, the complication rate was unacceptable and thus the concentration was subsequently reduced to 4%. The instillation of 4% formalin into the rectum therefore seemed a logical extension of the experience gained in treating hemorrhagic cystitis. In a report of 16 patients with radiation-induced hemorrhagic proctitis requiring transfusion, Saclarides et al.[23] instilled a 500-ml solution of 4% formalin into the rectum in 50-ml aliquots. Each aliquot was kept in contact with the rectal mucosa for approximately 30 seconds. After each aliquot, the formalin was aspirated and the rectal vault irrigated with saline. In between instillation of the aliquots, close attention was paid to rinsing the perineum in order to avoid any caustic injury to the anal canal or skin. Care was taken to avoid dilatation or traumatizing the anal canal in order to avoid anal fissures. In 12 of the 16 patients, bleeding stopped after single formalin instillation, while in three further patients the bleeding was considerably reduced; one patient required three treatments before the bleeding stopped. The only complications were in four patients who developed significant postoperative anal pain due to fissures. One patient reported persistent tenesmus and an increased number of stools, presumably due to reduced fecal capacity. The fissures of two of these four patients healed within 1 month; one healed more slowly and one persisted until the time of the patient's death from disseminated prostate cancer.

Despite the success of formalin, there have been concerns regarding its possible detrimental effect on rectal function. To evaluate this concern, we randomized 15 mongrel dogs weighing 50–60 lbs (23–27 kg) into five experimental groups according to time from formalin treatment: control, acute, 1 week, 2 weeks, and 4 weeks.[24] Formalin was instilled into the canine rectal vault using the method described above. Rectal compliance using a closed manometric system was assessed before and after formalin instillation at the designated time intervals. Serum formalin metabolites were determined at times 0, 0.5, 1, and 3 hours. A segment of rectal wall was then analyzed for collagen content, mucosal injury, and blood vessel density. Serum formalin levels peaked within 30 minutes, returning to baseline by 3 hours. With the exception of one dog, toxic levels were not reached at any time during the study. No dogs experienced sepsis, fever or altered gastrointestinal function. Dogs studied during the acute phase and at 1 week showed mild, diffuse proctitis and mucosal slough, which were absent at both 2 and 4 weeks; rectal compliance and collagen content were unchanged. The early decrease in mucosal blood vessels did not persist over time.

The formalin treatments have traditionally been administered in the operating room and have involved a one-night stay in the hospital. We have not chosen to undertake this technique as an outpatient procedure because of concerns regarding disposal of the toxic chemical once it is aspirated from the rectum and ventilation of a closed office space. Theoretically, a formalin-soaked cotton-tipped applicator could be placed through a rigid proctoscope and placed on the area of concern. However, in our experience, most cases of radiation proctitis have involved a diffuse area of the rectal mucosa and anastomosed to the dentate line. This pouch provides a neorectal segment with intact, intrinsic and extrinsic nerve and lymphovascular supply. Observations in two patients so treated demonstrated a 'good' quality evacuation pattern with 'good' neorectal tolerance volumes, compliance, and anal manometry. Faucheron *et al.*[35] reported their results using Soave's procedure as a final sphincter-saving solution for radiation-induced rectal pathology. Between January 1978 and July 1994, 30 consecutive patients underwent this operation as a final attempt to restore coloanal continuity. The mean follow-up was 4.2 years and early complications included postoperative hemorrhage and small bowel obstruction, and four patients developed pelvic or perianal sepsis. Three patients developed anastomotic strictures, which were treated with dilatation. Continence was described as normal in 19 of 23 evaluable patients.

The addition of a colonic J-pouch improves functional results because of the increased storage capacity of the neorectum. The benefit of the addition of a colonic J-pouch to a restorative proctectomy and coloanal anastomosis has been demonstrated in both retrospective and prospective randomized trials.[36–39] Alternatively, a segment of vascularized sigmoid colon graft may be used to separate the rectal and vaginal walls. This technique, also known as the Bricker–Johnston colonic patch, does not mandate resection of the diseased rectum and, as such, an extensive pelvic dissection with its potential for significant bleeding is avoided. Through a transabdominal approach, the rectum and vagina are separated and normal proximal colon is mobilized and advanced into the pelvis. The diseased rectum is longitudinally divided and the proximal colon is sutured to the open, diseased rectum; a proximal colostomy is then fashioned. This normal proximal bowel serves to increase the storage capability of the rectum and thereby improve function. A variation of this onlay patch technique involves division of the rectosigmoid junction followed by suturing of the open end of the distal sigmoid stump to the debrided edges of the fistular opening in the rectum. A loop is thereby created and evacuation of stool is accomplished initially by an end sigmoid colostomy. After healing has occurred, this colostomy is then mobilized and sutured to the pelvic loop of bowel.[40,41] The disadvantage of the Bricker–Johnston technique is that the diseased rectum is left in place and used for suturing. Experience with the Bricker–Johnston modifications is limited and the technique may not confer any advantage over the traditional coloanal anastomosis procedure with or without construction of a colonic J-pouch.

## CONCLUSION

Although most patients experience alteration in gastrointestinal and rectal function during pelvic radiation therapy, fortunately fewer experience long-term side effects. Treatment of the patient who has sustained a rectal injury must be individualized, taking into consideration patient factors such as overall medical health and rectal function. First and foremost, recurrent cancer must be excluded with endoscopy and biopsy of any suspicious lesions. Before embarking on any restorative procedures, disseminated disease must be excluded. Radiation-induced hemorrhagic proctitis can be successfully treated with the instillation of rectal formalin. Endoscopic attempts at laser ablation frequently require multiple sessions to produce a noticeable effect. Isolated rectovaginal fistulas without significant proctitis or loss of rectal compliance can be treated with transanal, transperineal, or transvaginal approaches. Although temporary fecal diversion is not routinely necessary, it should be considered for large fistulas or for patients who have previously undergone unsuccessful attempts at repair. Fistulas located in the middle and upper two-thirds of the rectum or those fistulas associated with significant proctitis and loss of compliance generally require either partial or complete proctectomy. Rectal stenosis is best managed by partial or complete proctectomy with colorectal or coloanal anastomosis with a colonic J-pouch. Alternative techniques with the Soave operation or the Bricker–Johnston onlay patch can be considered; however, these operations confer little, if any, benefit over the above-mentioned techniques.

## REFERENCES

1   Perez CA, Lee HK, Georgious A *et al.* Technical factors affecting morbidity in definitive irradiation for localized carcinoma of the prostate. *Int J Radiat Oncol Biol Phys* 1994;28:811–819

2   Schultheiss TE, Lee WR, Hung MA *et al.* Late GI and GU complications in the treatment of prostate cancer. *Int J Radiat Oncol Biol Phys* 1997;37:3–11

3   Hu K, Wallner K. Clinical course of rectal bleeding following I-125 prostate brachytherapy. *Int J Radiat Oncol Biol Phys* 1998;41:263–265

4   Perez CA, Grigsby PW, Camel HM *et al.* Irradiation alone or combined with surgery in stage IB, IIA, and IIB carcinoma of uterine cervix: update of a nonrandomized comparison. *Int J Radiat Oncol Biol Phys* 1995;31:703–716

5   Uno T, Itami J, Aruga M *et al.* High dose rate brachytherapy for carcinoma of the cervix: risk factors for late rectal complications. *Int J Radiat Oncol Biol Phys* 1998;40:615–621

6   Jereczek-Fossa B, Jassem J, Nowak R *et al.* Late complications after postoperative radiotherapy in endometrial cancer: analysis of 317 consecutive cases with application of linear-quadratic model. *Int J Radiat Oncol Biol Phys* 1998;**41**: 329–338

7   Allal AS, Mermillod B, Roth AD *et al.* Impact of clinical and therapeutic factors on major late complications after radiotherapy with or without concomitant chemotherapy for anal carcinoma. *Int J Radiat Oncol Biol Phys* 1997;**39**:1099–1105

8   Peiffert D, Bey P, Pernot M *et al.* Conservative treatment by irradiation of epidermoid carcinomas of the anal margin. *Int J Radiat Oncol Biol Phys* 1997; **39**:57–66

9   Montana GS, Anscher MS, Mansbach CM II *et al.* Topical application of WR-2721 to prevent radiation-induced proctosigmoiditis: a phase I/II trial. *Cancer* 1992;**69**: 2826–2830

10  Mitsuhashi N, Takahashi I, Takahashi M *et al.* Clinical study of radioprotective effects of amifostine (YM-08310, WR-2721) on long-term outcome for patients with cervical cancer. *Int J Radiat Oncol Biol Phys* 1993;**26**:407–411

11  Resbeut M, Marteau P, Cowen D *et al.* A randomized double blind placebo controlled multicenter study of mesalazine for the prevention of acute radiation enteritis. *Radiother Oncol* 1997;**44**:59–63

12  Farrell CL, Bready JV, Rex KL *et al.* Keratinocyte growth factor protects mice from chemotherapy and radiation-induced gastrointestinal injury and mortality. *Cancer Res* 1998;**58**:933–939

13  Talley NA, Chen F, King D *et al.* Short-chain fatty acids in the treatment of radiation proctitis: a randomized, double-blind placebo-controlled, cross-over pilot trial. *Dis Colon Rectum* 1997;**40**:1046–1050

14  Henriksson R, Franzen L, Littbrand B. Effects of sucralfate on acute and late bowel discomfort following radiotherapy of pelvic cancer. *J Clin Oncol* 1992;**10**: 969–975

15  O'Brien PC, Franklin CI, Dear KB *et al.* A phase III double-blind randomized study of rectal sucralfate suspension in the prevention of acute radiation proctitis. *Radiother Oncol* 1997;**45**:117–123

16  Delaney G, Fisher R, Hook C *et al.* Sucralfate cream in the management of moist desquamation during radiotherapy. *Australas Radiol* 1997;**41**:270–275

17  Warren DC, Feehan P, Slade JB *et al.* Chronic radiation proctitis treated with hyperbaric oxygen. *Undersea Hyperb Med* 1997;**24**:181–184

18  Woo TC, Joseph D, Oxer H. Hyperbaric oxygen treatment for radiation proctitis. *Int J Radiat Oncol Biol Phys* 1997;**38**:619–622

19  Favre C, Ventura A, Nardi M *et al.* Hyperbaric oxygen therapy in a case of post-total body irradiation colitis. *Bone Marrow Transplant* 1998;**21**:519–520

20  Barbatzas C, Spencer GM, Thorpe SM *et al.* Nd:YAG laser treatment for bleeding from radiation proctitis. *Endoscopy* 1996;**28**:497–500

21  Leuchter RS, Petrilli ES, Dwyer RM *et al.* Nd:YAG laser therapy of rectosigmoid bleeding due to radiation injury. *Obstet Gynecol* 1982;**59**(suppl 6):65S–67S

22  Taylor JG, DiSario JA, Buchi KN. Argon laser therapy for hemorrhagic radiation proctitis: long-term results. *Gastrointest Endosc* 1993;**39**:641–644

23 Saclarides TJ, King DG, Franklin JL *et al*. Formalin instillation for refractory radiation-induced hemorrhagic proctitis. Report of 16 patients. *Dis Colon Rectum* 1996;**39**:196–199

24 Myers JA, Hollinger EF, Mall JW *et al*. Mechanical, histologic, and biochemical effects of canine rectal formalin instillation. *Dis Colon Rectum* 1998;**41**:153–158

25 Rius J, Nessim A, Nogueras JJ, Wexner SD. Gracilis transposition in complicated perineal fistula and unhealed perineal wounds in Crohn's disease. *Eur J Surg* 2000; **166**:218–222

26 Rothenberger DA, Christenson CE, Balcos EG *et al*. Endorectal advancement flap for treatment of simple rectovaginal fistula. *Dis Colon Rectum* 1982;**25**: 297–300

27 Nessim A, Wexner SD, Agachan F *et al*. Is bowel confinement necessary after anorectal constructive surgery? A prospective randomized surgeon blinded trial. *Dis Colon Rectum* 1999;**42**:16–23

28 Lowry AC, Thorson AG, Rothenberger DA *et al*. Repair of simple rectovaginal fistulas. Influence of previous repairs. *Dis Colon Rectum* 1988;**31**:676–678

29 Hudson CN. Rectovaginal fistula: Vaginal repair. In: Fielding LP, Goldberg SM (eds) *Rob and Smith's Operative Surgery: Surgery of the Colon, Rectum and Anus*, 5th edn. Lippincott, Williams & Wilkins, Philadelphia, 1993;855

30 Turnbull Jr RB, Cuthbertson A. Abdominorectal pull-through resection for cancer and for Hirschsprung's disease. *Cleveland Clin Q* 1961;**28**:109–115

31 Kirwan WO, Turnbull Jr RB, Fazio VW *et al*. Pullthrough operation with delayed anastomosis for rectal cancer. *Br J Surg* 1978;**65**:695–698

32 Parks AG, Allen CL, Frank JD *et al*. A method of treating post-irradiation rectovaginal fistulas. *Br J Surg* 1978;**65**:417–421

33 Panis Y, Perrin H, Poupard B *et al*. Colonal anastomosis for benign lesions: long term functional results in 11 patients. *Eur J Surg* 1996;**162**:555–559

34 von Flue MO, Degen LP, Beglinger C *et al*. The ileocecal reservoir for rectal replacement in complicated radiation proctitis. *Am J Surg* 1996;**172**:335–340

35 Faucheron JL, Rosso R, Tiret E *et al*. Soave's procedure: the final sphincter-saving solution for iatrogenic rectal lesions. *Br J Surg* 1998;**85**:962–964

36 Hallbook O, Pahlman L, Krog M, Wexner SD, Sjodahl R. Randomized comparison of straight and colonic J pouch anastomosis after low anterior resection. *Ann Surg* 1996;**224**:58–65

37 Joo JS, Latulippe JF, Alabaz O, Weiss EG, Nogueras JJ, Wexner SD. Long term functional evaluation of straight coloanal anastomosis and colonic J pouch. Is the functional superiority of colonic J pouch sustained? *Dis Colon Rectum* 1998;**41**: 740–746

38 Parc R, Tiret E, Frileux P, Moszkowski E, Loygue J. Resection and colo-anal anastomosis with colonic reservoir in colorectal cancer. *Br J Surg* 1986;**73**:139–141

39 Seow-Choen F, Goh HS. Prospective, randomized trial comparing J colonic pouch and anastomosis and straight coloanal reconstruction. *Br J Surg* 1995;**82**:608–610

40 Bricker EM, Johnston WD. Repair of postirradiation rectovaginal fistula and stricture. *Surg Gynecol Obstet* 1979;**148**:499–506

41 Bricker EM, Johnston WD, Patwardhan RV. Repair of postirradiation damage to colorectum: a progress report. *Ann Surg* 1981;**193**:555–564

# Index